Personal

YOUR GUIDE TO UNDERSTANDING AND DEALING WITH TYPE 2 DIABETES

What You Need to Know

Dr Keith Souter

Manjul Publishing House

First published in India by

MANJUL

Manjul Publishing House

Corporate and Editorial Office

• 2nd Floor, Usha Preet Complex, 42 Malviya Nagar, Bhopal 462 003 - India

Sales and Marketing Office

• 7/32, Ground Floor, Ansari Road, Daryaganj, New Delhi 110 002 - India

Website: www.manjulindia.com

Distribution Centres

Ahmedabad, Bengaluru, Bhopal, Kolkata, Chennai,
Hyderabad, Mumbai, New Delhi, Pune

YOUR GUIDE TO UNDERSTANDING AND DEALING WITH TYPE 2 DIABETES by Dr Keith Souter

This edition first published in India in 2016
by arrangement with Summersdale Publishers Ltd.

ISBN 978-81-8322-718-6

Printed and bound in India by Manipal Technologies Ltd., Manipal

Disclaimer

Every effort has been made to ensure that the information in this book is accurate and current at the time of publication. The author and the publisher cannot accept responsibility for any misuse or misunderstanding of any information contained herein, or any loss, damage or injury, be it health, financial or otherwise, suffered by any individual or group acting upon or relying on information contained herein. None of the opinions or suggestions in this book are intended to replace medical opinion. If you have concerns about your health, please seek professional advice.

In memory of my mother, Mollie Anne McDonald Souter, who lived well with her Type 2 diabetes for many years

Acknowledgements

I would like to thank Isabel Atherton, my wonderful agent at Creative Authors for helping to bring another book in this series to fruition. Thanks also to Claire Plimmer at Summersdale who commissioned this and the previous titles, and to Anna Martin who has skilfully guided it through the various stages towards publication. Thanks to Ellie Clarke for doing the initial edit to knock the rough edges off the manuscript and to Lyn Coutts my copy-editor for smoothing it still further. I am grateful for the many helpful suggestions that have been made at every stage, which have helped to make it a more readable and accessible book.

It has been another enjoyable experience working with Summersdale Publishers.

Keith Souter

Contents

Introduction

If you have recently been diagnosed with Type 2 diabetes, you may be thinking that you have been given bad news. You may think life as you have enjoyed it is at an end and that you are faced with a future of deterioration. This does not have to be the case at all. Type 2 diabetes is a condition to take seriously, but the diagnosis gives you the opportunity to get it under control and to reduce your risk of developing complications. Indeed, control it well and you will probably feel better than you have done for some time.

You may not, in fact, have been diagnosed with the condition, but been told that you have pre-diabetes. This means that you are at risk of developing it, but as yet you have not done so. The very good news is that you can reverse that risk and prevent yourself from developing Type 2 diabetes.

Diabetes is a condition that is increasing in incidence every year around the globe. It is linked with rising obesity levels, greater inactivity and the consumption of a diet that frankly predisposes people to develop diabetes.

As we shall see in Chapter 1 (*An overview of diabetes*) diabetes mellitus is a lifelong disorder of carbohydrate metabolism that occurs when the pancreas does not produce enough insulin, or when the body does not respond to its own insulin. While I am going to consider the different types, the overall emphasis of the book is on understanding and dealing with Type 2 diabetes.

The book falls naturally into two parts. Part 1 is about understanding Type 2 diabetes, beginning with some background information about the way the body's metabolism works and how the body handles glucose. Then we shall look at how things can go wrong and what sort of complications can occur. This is important, because Type 2 diabetes can affect many of the body's systems, particularly the circulation and heart, the eyes, the kidneys and the nervous system. You need to know about all of these in order to reduce your risk of developing such complications.

Part 2 will look at how diabetes is diagnosed and how you and your doctor can keep it under control. We will look at the tests and investigations you should have, and we will look at the way that diet, exercise and possibly drugs can maximise your health.

The diagnosis is not bad news; it is a warning that things are not working as they should, and by altering lifestyle and developing a positive attitude towards the condition and your future, you can live well with your Type 2 diabetes.

Part One

UNDERSTANDING TYPE 2 DIABETES

Type 2 diabetes does not always produce the common symptoms, such as increased thirst. This is very important, because many people with Type 2 diabetes have no symptoms at all, or are not particularly bothered by them for years. They may not know that they have diabetes until they have a blood-glucose test done on routine examination at their doctor's surgery. Because of this tendency for the condition to smoulder on unrecognised, if you believe that you are at risk of developing it, you should have a blood test.

Chapter 1

An overview of diabetes

Diabetes mellitus is a lifelong disorder of carbohydrate metabolism that occurs when the pancreas does not produce enough insulin or when the tissues do not respond to the body's own insulin.

The characteristic feature of diabetes in an undiagnosed or untreated form is excess thirst and increased tendency to pass urine. This is the result of raised blood-glucose levels. Over time this can lead to serious damage to various body systems.

Common symptoms of diabetes

- Increased thirst
- Increased frequency of urination, especially at night
- Excessive tiredness
- Weight loss and loss of muscle bulk
- Itching around the genitals or frequent episodes of thrush
- Wounds or cuts are slow to heal
- Blurred vision, as a result of the lens of the eyes becoming dry

Types of diabetes

There are two main types of diabetes, which make up the vast majority of cases. They share the name diabetes mellitus, but each type has its own features, causes and indicated treatments.

Both types affect the blood-glucose levels and both produce complications unless they are adequately treated. These complications can significantly impair health and even lead to early death.

Type 1 diabetes

This is characterised by lack of insulin production. It used to be called juvenile onset diabetes or insulin dependent diabetes. This was because it tended to occur in children and young adults. It requires treatment with insulin.

It is an autoimmune condition in which the immune system attacks the insulin-producing cells in the pancreas. There is therefore a deficiency of insulin and the individual will have to take insulin injections for the rest of his or her life. It is not possible at this stage in time to prevent Type 1 diabetes from developing. Type 1 diabetes accounts for about ten per cent of all diabetes cases worldwide.

Type 2 diabetes

This is characterised by ineffective response to the body's own insulin.

It used to be called maturity onset diabetes, or insulin independent diabetes. This was because it tended to occur in adults who are overweight. The treatment usually involves dietary control and possibly oral hypoglycaemic drugs to lower the blood-glucose.

It is perfectly possible to prevent Type 2 diabetes. Type 2 diabetes accounts for about 90 per cent of all diabetes cases worldwide.

Gestational diabetes

This is diabetes that starts during pregnancy and goes away at the end of the pregnancy. It is usually discovered in the middle trimester of pregnancy.

Why we use the terms Type 1 and Type 2

The main reason why the older names are no longer used is simply because we are seeing increasing incidence of the following diabetes variants around the world. We see Type 1 developing in adults and we see Type 2 developing in children. In some countries, Type 2 accounts for almost half of newly diagnosed diabetes in children and adults.

OTHER LESS COMMON TYPES OF DIABETES

There are other less common types of diabetes. Cumulatively, they account for a mere two per cent of diabetes cases.

- MODY (maturity-onset diabetes of youth) – this is caused as a result of mutations affecting beta cells of the islets of Langerhans, which are the insulin-producing cells in the pancreas. (See Chapter 3: *So what happens in diabetes?*)
- Neonatal hypoglycaemia – a type of diabetes that occurs before the age of six months and is usually due to a genetic mutation.
- Diabetes as part of other endocrine (hormonal) diseases, for example: Cushing's syndrome, acromegaly and thyrotoxicosis.

- Pancreatic disease – for example: cystic fibrosis (a disorder in which the lungs and digestive system get clogged with sticky mucus) and haemochromatosis (a disorder in which the body stores excess iron).
- Iatrogenic diabetes – meaning 'doctor-induced' from long-term steroid drug use or HIV drug treatment, for example.

Complications of diabetes

There are several possible complications from diabetes that may be divided into groups.

- Metabolic – problems with sugar levels, either from the condition or its treatment. The condition also affects protein and fat metabolism.
- Vascular – these can be subdivided into:
    1. Macro-vascular – disease of large blood vessels, for example: coronary arteries (angina and heart attacks), peripheral arteries (intermittent claudication) and cerebral arteries (strokes).
    2. Micro-vascular – disease of small blood vessels, for example: diabetic retinopathy (blood vessels in the retinae of the eyes), nephropathy (blood vessels in the kidneys) and neuropathy (blood vessels to the small tissues and the nerves).
- Immune impairment – making diabetics more susceptible to infections

- Cataracts and other eye problems
- Erectile dysfunction and loss of libido
- Foot and joint problems
- Skin problems

Diabetes is a leading cause of blindness, amputation and kidney failure.

Women who are already diabetic before they conceive a child are five times more likely to have babies with congenital heart disease than women without diabetes.

Babies born to women who develop gestational diabetes do not have the same risk because the condition tends to occur in the middle trimester after the baby's heart and organs have developed.

Life expectancy

Diabetes is a serious condition that can lead to early death if it is not carefully managed.

According to Diabetes UK, the life expectancy on average is reduced by:

- more than 20 years for people with Type 1 diabetes.
- up to ten years for people with Type 2 diabetes.

With good control of the diabetes, however, there is normal life expectancy.

KEY POINT

Cardiovascular disease, including heart attacks and strokes accounts for 50–80 per cent of deaths in people with diabetes.

Pre-diabetes

This is a very important condition. It is when the blood-glucose level is higher than normal, but not high enough to be diagnosed as diabetes. It is a state that increases the risk of diabetes.

It is estimated that there are around seven million people in the UK with pre-diabetes. The good news is that with alteration of lifestyle consisting of a healthy diet, regular physical activity, maintaining a normal body weight and avoiding tobacco use Type 2 diabetes can be avoided.

Some risk factors for diabetes

There are a number of factors that increase the risk of diabetes.

Genetic tendency

The likelihood of developing Type 2 diabetes is also influenced by genetics and environmental factors. Research[1] has shown that if:

- either parent has Type 2 diabetes, the risk of inheritance of Type 2 diabetes is 15 per cent.

- both parents have Type 2 diabetes, the risk of inheritance of Type 2 diabetes is 75 per cent.

Ethnicity

A lot of attention has been paid to changes in lifestyle, as many countries have adopted Western diets, with drastic increase in diabetes and increased incidence of heart disease and stroke. This has been particularly apparent in certain ethnic groups, such as some Native Americans and indigenous Australians.

The risk of diabetes is increased for some ethnic groups and reduced for others. Type 2 diabetes is six times more prevalent in people of South Asian ancestry[2] and three times more likely to occur in people of African and Afro-Caribbean ancestry.

Obesity and diabetes

There seems to be a clear link between obesity and diabetes. It has been observed that as the incidence of obesity rises, so too does the incidence of diabetes.

In Japan, the incidence of diabetes is relatively low. However, among Japanese people who emigrated to the USA and adopted a Western lifestyle and diet, the incidence of both obesity and diabetes rose. Interestingly, in sumo wrestlers in Japan, who have to maintain body bulk in order to compete in this traditional sport, diabetes rates are significantly above normal.

KEY POINTS

Risk factors for Type 2 diabetes include:

- large waist (over 94 centimetres for men and 80 centimetres for women) or being overweight.
- being of African, Afro–Caribbean or South Asian origin.
- a family history of the condition.
- being over 40 years old, or over 25 if of African, Afro-Caribbean or South Asian origin, or from an ethnic minority group.

Diabetes around the world

Diabetes mellitus is an important condition for both the individual and for society. It is important to the individual because it can affect his or her overall health. It predisposes people to other conditions and has many potential complications. If it is poorly controlled it can lead to early death.

The number of people suffering from diabetes is increasing every year. This seems to be the result of social changes in dietary habits with overconsumption of energy-rich foods, rising levels of obesity and more sedentary lifestyles.

Diabetes throws a significant load on the heath resources of all countries and, since so many people who are diagnosed with it are of working age, it can have a huge impact on a country's economy.

Most deaths are likely to take place in countries with limited resources where there are not facilities for renal dialysis or complex surgery. Indeed, insulin is not available in many of the poorest countries. This accounts for the high mortality rates in those countries.

About 80 per cent of all people with diabetes live in the poorest countries. By comparison, around 80 per cent of the money spent on diabetes care occurs in the richest countries.

KEY POINTS

- Globally, there are about 347 million people with diabetes – this is a prevalence of just under five per cent of the world's population.[3]
- The International Diabetes Federation state that the countries with the greatest numbers of diabetics are respectively China, India, USA, Russia and Brazil.
- The International Diabetes Federation states that the countries with the highest prevalence rates are Saudi Arabia, Nauru and Mauritius.
- More than 80 per cent of diabetic deaths occur in low- and middle-income countries.[4]
- The World Health Organization (WHO) predicts that diabetes deaths will double between 2005 and 2030.
- WHO predicts that diabetes will become the seventh leading cause of death in the world by 2030.

Note: Prevalence means the number of people with a specific condition at a specified time divided by the total population.

UK situation

The UK has a population of 63 million, the third largest in the European Union.[5] According to the charity Diabetes UK, there are around 850,000 people in the UK who have undiagnosed diabetes.

KEY POINTS

- Currently there are over 3.1 million people aged 16 or over with diabetes in the UK.
- By 2030 it is predicted that there will be over 4.6 million people aged 16 or over with diabetes in the UK.
- Six per cent of adults have diabetes.
- 85–90 per cent of all diabetics have Type 2 diabetes.
- Ten per cent of all diabetics have Type 1 diabetes.
- Two to five in every 100 women giving birth in England and Wales develops gestational diabetes.

Cost

Diabetes UK estimates that around ten per cent of the NHS annual budget is used to fund treatment of diabetes, equating to about £9 billion per year.

Diabetes can affect anyone

Having diabetes should not stop you from enjoying life and being successful in your chosen field.

- Elvis Presley – the king of rock 'n' roll had diabetes.
- Queen Hatshepsut – a pharaoh of ancient Egypt who apparently had diabetes.
- Johnny Cash – the singer, had diabetes.

- George Lucas – the producer of *Star Wars* has Type 2 diabetes.
- Gary Hall – the Olympic swimmer has Type 1 diabetes.
- Sir Steve Redgrave – multiple Olympic Gold rower has Type 1 diabetes.
- Halle Berry – a movie star who has diabetes (originally diagnosed Type 1, but re-diagnosed Type 2).

Chapter 2

'The honey-sweet siphon' – the history of diabetes

Medical writers have been aware of this condition for at least 4,000 years. Its nature and its cause, however, remained a mystery for centuries.

The fact that writers in different cultures observed and advised about this condition makes it clear that diabetes has affected people around the world throughout history. As we will see in this chapter, it is not a condition restricted to the modern world. Having said that, contemporary lifestyles may be making diabetes more common than it was in the past.

Ancient Egypt – first observations

In 1862, Edwin Smith, a young amateur Egyptologist and adventurer, purchased two papyri in Luxor. It is unclear from whom he bought them, but it is said that they had been found between the legs of a mummy in the El-Asasif area of the Theban necropolis on the other side of the Nile from Luxor.

Both these papyri dated to about 1,534 BCE, but were thought to be copies of far older texts. One became known as the Edwin Smith papyrus and is the oldest known surgical text in the world. The other was eventually purchased by German Egyptologist Georg Ebers in 1872. This papyrus is a medical text outlining the state of Egyptian knowledge about medicine and the treatment of over 700 afflictions.

The Ebers papyrus is thought to have been written by a physician called Hesy-Ra, who mentions several types of urinary problem, some of which almost certainly refer to urinary infections like cystitis, where the main symptom is frequent micturition, or passage of urine. He makes a distinction between the frequent passage of urine with pain (which would have been from urinary infections) and the frequent passage of a lot of urine without pain, which we call polyuria. The latter is almost certainly a description of diabetes. The treatment advised by Hesy-Ra included a liquid extract of bones together with grain, grit, wheat, green lead and earth. Unfortunately, it is unlikely that the treatment would have had any beneficial effect.

Ancient India – the two different types of diabetes

The Indian surgeon and physician Sushruta (600–501 BCE) wrote a textbook called *Sushruta-samhita*, which means Sushruta's compendium. In it he details 650 drugs used by doctors of his time. In addition, he detailed many operations using 42 surgical techniques and over 120 surgical instruments. He gave instructions on how to surgically repair the nose (cutting off the nose being the penalty for adultery and other transgressions) and also how to do a lithotomy, the operation to remove urinary stones. He is recognised as the father of plastic surgery.

He describes the symptoms of diabetes, which he called *madhumeh*, to describe the sweetness and stickiness of the patient's urine. *Madu* is used in several Indo-Aryan languages to mean honey or sweet.

Another Indian physician called Charaka, who is thought to have flourished sometime between the second century BCE and the second century CE, refined Sushruta's observations. He wrote the *Charaka-samhita*, meaning Charaka's compendium, and in it differentiates between two types of diabetics. One group, who were thin and young and another group who were older and fatter. He also noted that the older group lived longer. This was the first attempt to divide diabetics into two groups, basically Type 1 and Type 2.

Remarkably, Charaka suggested a test: if the urine of such a patient was poured near an anthill it would attract ants!

Ancient Greece – diabetes

Aretaeus of Cappadocia first used the word 'diabetes' in the second century CE to indicate this condition. The word was derived from *dia* meaning 'through' and *betes* meaning 'passing', likening the passing through of urine to a siphon action. He also described the characteristic of the disease, which causes 'a melting down of the flesh and limbs into the urine.' He thought that it was a disorder of kidney function.

Claudius Galenus of Pergamum (*circa* 130–200 CE) was a famous second-century Greek physician practising in the Roman Empire. He described the excessive passage of urine, which he called *diarrhoea urinosa*, and the extreme thirst as *dipsakos*.

Ancient China and Japan

The sweetness of the urine of diabetics was noted by the Chinese physician Chen Chuan in the seventh century CE. At about the same time the Japanese physician Li Hsuan noted that the sweet urine of these patients would attract dogs. He also noted that diabetic patients were more likely to develop infections, including boils and sores and a respiratory disorder that was like tuberculosis.

Both Chen Chuan and Li Hsuan recommended that it should be treated by abstinence from sex and from wine and the avoidance of salty food, which would make the thirst worse. This is perfectly logical, of course, but focusing on the avoidance of sugar and sweets would have been more effective.

Arabic medicine

In the tenth century CE, the great Persian polymath known as Avicenna (980–1037 CE) pushed the frontiers of medicine on several fronts.

An astute clinician, he wrote that diabetes was associated with two specific complications. Firstly, there was a 'fall down' of sexual function. Secondly, people with this condition were prone to develop gangrene of their extremities. As we shall see later in this book, these are definite complications.

He also improved the method of giving medication by coating his pills in silver or gold leaf. In an age of alchemy, precious metals were thought to enhance the effectiveness of medicines. This also reduced the bitter taste of many medicines.

For diabetes, he advocated a mixture of herbs including lupin, fenugreek and zedoary (white turmeric) seeds. These do, in fact, have mild hypoglycaemic effects (they lower blood-sugar) so they would have had some positive consequence.

The Renaissance – discoveries about the cause and the first effective treatment

This period of time saw an explosion in science, philosophy, art and literature.

Doctors like William Harvey (1578–1657) studied anatomy and started to give an explanation for the way that the body worked. He was a physician and anatomist who fought in the English Civil War and who was court physician to three kings of England. After graduating from Cambridge University, he went to study medicine and anatomy at the University of Padua in Italy. In 1616 he announced his discovery of the circulation of the blood, and in 1628 he published his work *Exercitatio Anatomica de Motu Cordis et Sanguinis in Animalibus* (*An Anatomical Exercise on the Motion of the Heart and Blood in Animals*). It was the most significant piece of medical research ever written and laid the foundation for the scientific study of medicine.

Dr Thomas Willis (1621–1675) was another anatomist who, like Harvey, was deeply interested in the body's blood supply. He published several books in the 1660s, the most significant being a work about the brain. In it he described the circle of blood vessels at the base of the brain, which were formed from major arteries travelling up the front of the neck to join with ones from the back of the neck to produce an arterial circle which gave off branches to supply blood to the various areas of the brain. This is called the Circle of Willis.

Dr Willis was also intrigued by diabetes. He referred to it as 'the pissing evil', but went on to state that diabetic urine was 'wonderfully sweet as if it were imbued with honey or sugar' since tasting patients' urine was an art that most physicians practiced in his day. He added the Latin word *mellitus*, meaning 'honey-sweet'. Hence, the name *diabetes mellitus* literally means the honey-sweet syphon, which effectively describes the symptoms of excessive urination of sweet urine.

Dr Thomas Sydenham (1624–1689) wrote a textbook *Observationes Medicae*, the major text for two centuries, in which he proposed that diabetes was not merely a disorder of the urinary system (as had been thought until then) but was in actuality a systemic disorder. This means that it affects many of the body's systems.

In 1776 Liverpool physician Dr Matthew Dobson performed a series of experiments and discovered that there was a sweet-tasting substance in both the urine and the blood serum of patients with diabetes. When he evaporated the urine and the blood serum he was able to identify that the sweetness was due to the presence of sugar.

In 1788 Dr Thomas Cawley performed post-mortem examinations on diabetic patients and noted that there were physical changes in the pancreas. He deduced that somehow this organ was involved in the development of the condition.

In 1797 a Scottish physician, Dr John Rollo, used the urine glucose test devised by Dr Dobson to show that diabetes could be treated by diet, which could reduce the sugar in the urine. He advocated a diet of animal food, 'plain blood puddings and fat and rancid meat', which was also low in vegetable matter. This meant basing the diet on meat and cutting out vegetables and bread. Effectively, he was recommending a high-protein, low-carbohydrate diet. This would certainly have helped his diabetic patients.

The nineteenth and twentieth centuries – the discoveries about the pancreas and insulin

In the Victorian era, doctors began to discover the nature of metabolism and the physiology of the pancreas.

The French physician Claude Bernard (1813–1878) studied rabbits and concluded that sugar was stored in the liver as a chemical called glycogen. He also discovered that the nervous system was involved in controlling blood-glucose concentrations.

Paul Langerhans (1847–1888), while studying for his doctorate in Berlin in 1869, noticed small clusters of cells within the pancreas. He was unaware of their function, however.

In 1889 in Strasbourg in Germany, Bernard Naunyn, Oscar Minowski and Joseph Freiherr von Mering removed the pancreas from dogs to ascertain whether this would have an effect on blood-sugar levels. The effect was to produce diabetes in the dogs, with increased thirst, excessive urination, wasting of muscles and ultimately, death. However, if instead of removing the pancreas they merely ligated (tied off) the pancreatic duct, this would prevent pancreatic juices from reaching the intestine. The dog would experience stomach problems, but it would not become diabetic.

These experiments proved that the pancreas was crucial in the metabolism of sugar and had an important role in diabetes. Yet somehow, something in the pancreas was still finding its way into the blood stream to control the blood-sugar. Clearly it was something that was passed directly to the blood stream rather than being passed into the intestines with the pancreatic juices.

Four years later in 1893 Edouard Laguesse (1861–1927) deduced that the cells that Langerhans had found in the pancreas were involved in sugar metabolism. He therefore called them the islets of Langerhans.

In 1909 Jean de Meyer isolated the hormone that lowered glucose levels from the islets of Langerhans. He called this hormone insulin, from the Latin *insula*, meaning island, because it had been produced from the islets of Langerhans.

The search for a treatment

In the 1920s, the Canadian doctor Frederick Banting (1891–1941) was working in Ontario. He had the idea that a lack of insulin could cause diabetes. Until then it had been impossible to extract insulin from the pancreas.

Working with Charles Best (1899–1978), a young biomedical scientist, Banting performed experiments on dogs to measure their blood- and urine-sugar levels. Their experiments were being supervised by Professor John MacLeod, who held the chair of physiology at the university. In 1921 Banting and Best managed to extract insulin and a year later they treated a young teenager, Leonard Thompson, who had diabetes mellitus, by giving him injections of insulin. The results were incredible, they had developed the first really effective treatment for severe diabetes and transformed the outlook for patients. Instead of facing a condition that could kill within days, it meant that diabetic patients could live a normal life, albeit necessitating regular injections.

From then on there was a need to obtain large amounts of insulin, which was done by extracting it from the pancreas of slaughtered cows and pigs. This is still done to produce respectively bovine and porcine insulin. They are chemically modified, of course, to make them resemble human insulin.

Banting and Macleod were awarded the Nobel Prize in Physiology or Medicine in 1923 for the discovery of insulin.

Insulin analysed and the development of Humulin

In 1928 the chemical structure of insulin was elucidated by Oskar Wintersteiner. He proved that it was a protein made up of amino acids.

In 1955 Frederick Sanger worked out the actual structure of insulin. He proposed that it was made up of two chains of proteins connected by a disulphide bond. For this he was awarded the 1958 Nobel Prize in Chemistry.

Sanger's work allowed a human insulin gene to be made, which could then be used to genetically engineer bacteria to produce large amounts of pure human insulin. This was called Humulin.

Oral hypoglycaemic agents

Having to have a daily injection of insulin takes a lot of getting used to, and it was found that not all diabetics needed insulin. It was known that there were two types of diabetes, and they were referred to initially as insulin dependent diabetes (or juvenile diabetes), which is now called Type 1 diabetes, and non-insulin dependent diabetes (or maturity-onset diabetes), now called Type 2 diabetes.

In 1942 the first oral hypoglycaemic agent (blood-sugar lowering drug) was produced by Marcel Janbon while working on a drug to treat typhoid fever. It took another ten years before Franke and Fuchs in Berlin introduced the sulphonylurea group of drugs as the first effective hypoglycaemic drugs in the treatment of diabetes.

The biguanide drugs (phenformin and then metformin) were then introduced, followed in the 1990s by the thiazolidenediones. We will be looking at all of these in Chapter 9 (*Drugs for Type 2 diabetes*).

Chapter 3

Metabolism and what goes wrong in diabetes

You may think it seems odd that having an excess of glucose, which is the body's main energy source, can be bad for you. Well, in order to understand why, we need to have a look at metabolism and the way that the body handles glucose.

Metabolism

This refers to the life-sustaining chemical reactions or transformations that occur within the cells of the body. The term comes from the Greek, meaning change or transform.

Thousands of these reactions take place at once in a never-ending series to keep the cells nourished, healthy and able to perform their work. Metabolism inside your cells never stops from the moment you are conceived until the time that you die. If metabolism stops, then death occurs.

Enzymes

The fuel that we take into our system as food is digested and broken down in the digestive tract by a number of specific enzymes. These are special molecules that catalyse or regulate specific reactions. Of these, there are particular enzymes that break proteins down to amino acids, others that break fats down to fatty acids, and still others that break carbohydrates down to simple sugars, such as glucose. These amino acids, fatty acids and sugars are absorbed into the blood and transported to the cells of the body. These are considered to be the building blocks of the body.

Inside the cells, different enzymes speed up and regulate all of the chemical reactions that are involved in metabolising the amino acids, fatty acids and sugars to release energy. The transformed substances can either be used in further metabolic reactions or they can be transferred to be stored in the cells of various body tissues. For example, glycogen can be stored in the liver and the muscles of the body, while fat is stored in adipose cells that make up the body's fat deposits. As we shall see, the metabolism of proteins, fats and carbohydrates is all linked, and it is all regulated in order to maintain balance in the cells, tissues, organs and fluids of the body.

A fine balancing act

In order to maintain this state of internal balance there are two types of metabolic process that go on in the cells.

Anabolism

These are reactions that build and store. They are responsible for helping new cells grow, build new tissues and store energy in a manner that it can be used when needed.

Anabolic reactions change the building block molecules into more complex protein, fat and carbohydrate molecules. To do this they use energy, thus:

- glycogenesis – the building of glycogen from glucose.
- glyconeogenesis – the generation of glucose from non-carbohydrate substances, such as pyruvate, lactate, glycerol and amino acids.
- lipogenesis – the building of triglyceride fats from fatty acids.

Catabolism

These reactions break down the building blocks into even simpler molecules, with the release of energy. They also use up the energy stores.

Waste products are formed as larger molecules are broken down in to simpler ones. These are released and removed from the body through the various excretory organs; the lungs, digestive tract, kidneys and skin.

Catabolic reactions end in 'lysis', which means breaking down. It comes from the Greek, meaning to unbind. Thus:

- lipolysis – breaking down fats into fatty acids
- proteolysis – breaking down proteins into amino acids
- glycolysis – breaking down glucose into pyruvate
- glycogenolysis – breaking down glycogen into glucose.

You can see some of these reactions and the way that they are potentially reversible in the simplified diagram of metabolism in Figure 1.

Figure 1:
Metabolism of fats, carbohydrates and proteins

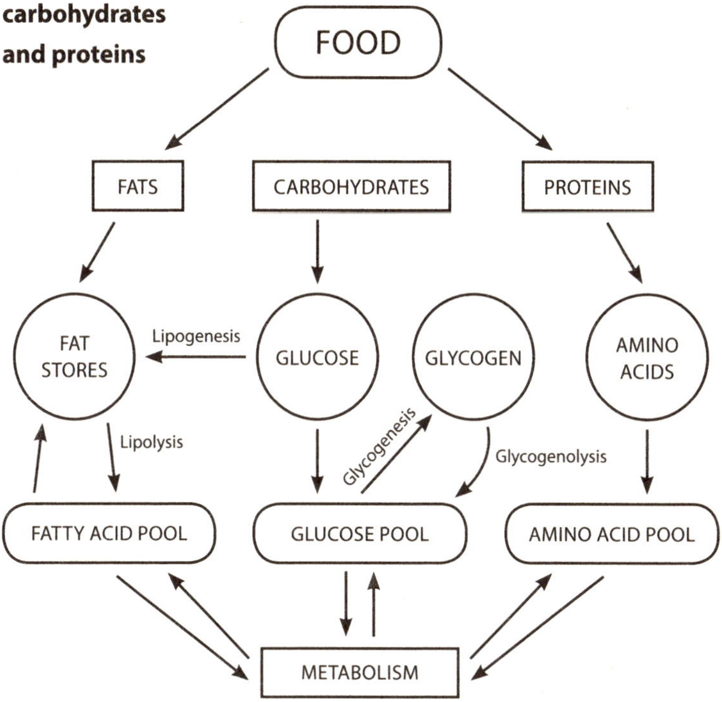

Normal glucose metabolism

The metabolism is regulated to produce a constant supply of glucose to the cells, rather than having extremes of highs and lows. If there is too much glucose it gets stored in another form, by being converted into the more complex molecule of glycogen. If there is insufficient, then stores of glycogen get broken down to produce enough glucose to fuel the reactions in the cells. There are balancing anabolic and catabolic reactions going on all the time to keep the glucose level steady.

Glycogenesis

Glucose molecules cannot be broken down further until they have been converted to another substance called glucose-6-phosphate. This reaction is catalysed by the enzyme hexokinase in cells. It is also catalysed by the enzyme glucokinase in the liver.

Once glucose has become glucose-6-phosphate it can be converted into glycogen, which is a molecule made up of long chains of glucose molecules. This is the form in which glucose is stored. It can be stored in the liver or in the muscles.

Glycolysis

Glucose-6-phosphate can undergo a catabolic reaction, a breaking down to produce another chemical called pyruvate. The pyruvate is then transformed into acetyl-coenzyme A. This is called glycolysis.

Acetyl-coenzyme A, usually abbreviated to acetyl-CoA, is an important molecule in metabolism because it can be used in both anabolic and catabolic reactions.

- The anabolic reaction, called lipogenesis, to produce fats.
- The catabolic reaction known as the Krebs cycle.

The Krebs cycle

This is one of the most important reactions in all metabolism. It is also called the citric acid cycle or the tricarboxylic acid cycle (the TCA cycle). It is the main energy-producing reaction that goes on in the cells. It is named after Hans Adolf Krebs who discovered, while working at Sheffield University in the UK, the sequence of reactions that take place in a continual cycle. He received the Nobel Prize in Physiology or Medicine for it in 1953.

The Krebs cycle needs the presence of oxygen. It results in the release of molecules of carbon dioxide and water and several 'packets' of energy as it goes through each cycle. The first step involves citric acid, hence one of the names it is given.

You can really think of it as a sort of hopper into which the building blocks formed from the breakdown of fats, proteins and carbohydrates are fed to produce energy.

The Krebs cycle effectively links up carbohydrate metabolism with fat and protein metabolism. Essentially, it takes in acetyl-CoA, which is manufactured from glucose and oxaloacetate, to form citric acid that is very high in energy.

The citric acid gradually loses energy and carbon dioxide. The carbon dioxide is a waste product, which is removed. The energy is collected as energy-carrying molecules, which produce adenosine triphosphate (ATP), which is used to power all sorts of other chemical reactions in the cells. There are several main steps in this cycle, which sees the six-carbon molecule reduced to a five-carbon molecule (when one carbon molecule of carbon dioxide is given off), then to a four-carbon molecule (when another one carbon molecule of carbon dioxide is released) – before again being built up to the six-carbon molecule of citric acid again, after the addition of more acetyl-CoA, which is a two-carbon molecule.

For our purposes we need not go into this in any further detail. Figure 2 illustrates the way in which some of these various metabolic processes, both anabolic and catabolic are inter-related. All you need to take away from this is the cyclical manner in which citric acid is broken down and then reconstructed, with the net release of packets of energy used to fuel the chemical reactions of metabolism.

Figure 2:
The Krebs cycle

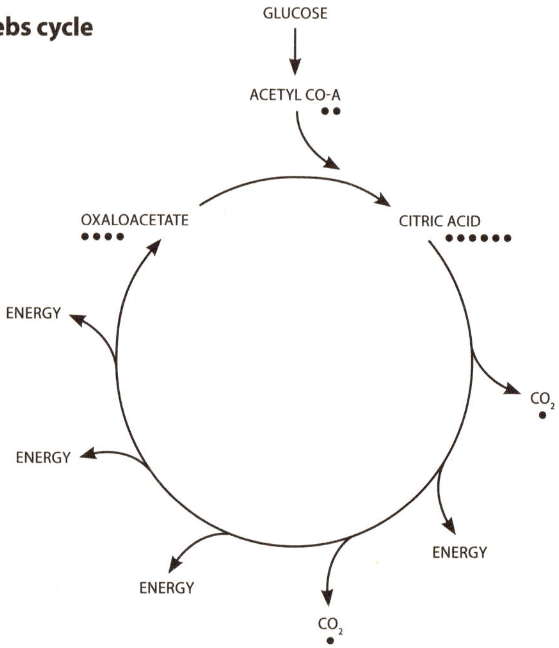

Glucose production

When there is an insufficient level of glucose, such as can happen when someone is fasting or vomiting and therefore taking in no food, then two processes can be used to increase the amount of glucose. One is anabolic and the other is catabolic. So, once again you can see how metabolism is a balancing act.

Glycogenolysis

This is the catabolic reaction that results in the breakdown of glycogen into glucose. As mentioned above, glycogen can be stored in the liver or in the muscles, so it can be released from there. The liver stores are the largest.

Gluconeogenesis

This is an anabolic reaction in which glucose is produced from either fatty acids or amino acids. Fatty acids are the building blocks of fats, while amino acids are the building blocks of protein.

The pancreas and the hormonal control of blood-glucose

The pancreas is a long, soft organ found just beneath the stomach, tucked inside the loop of the duodenum. The stomach passes its food contents into the duodenum, which is the first part of the small intestine. The pancreas is a remarkable organ that has a role in two different types of organ systems. These are the exocrine and the endocrine systems.

The exocrine system includes all the organs of the body that release their contents through a duct. It includes the sweat glands that lubricate the skin and the salivary glands that produce saliva. The bulk of the pancreas has exocrine functions and produces digestive enzymes, which are secreted into the duodenum via the pancreatic duct.

The endocrine system includes the organs that produce hormones, which are pumped directly into the bloodstream, rather than through a duct. They are sometimes referred to as the ductless glands. These include the pituitary, thyroid and adrenal glands and the testes and ovaries.

The islets of Langerhans are small areas found in the pancreas that have this endocrine function. They produce two hormones that regulate the blood-glucose level in the body.

Figure 3:
The pancreas and the cells of the islets of Langerhans

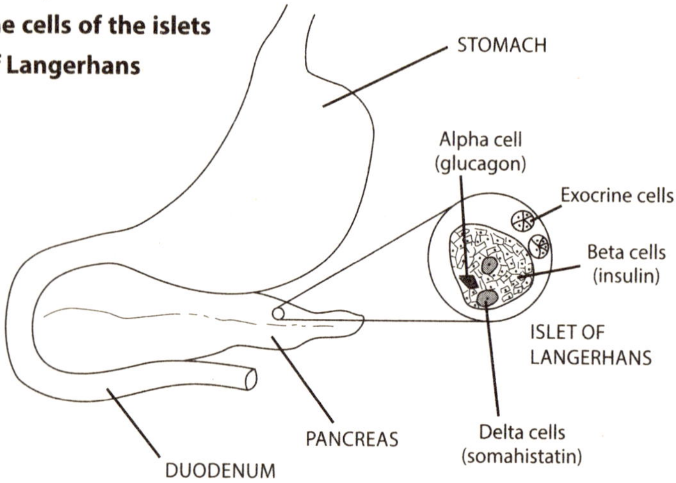

Glucagon and insulin

The islets of Langerhans are composed of alpha, beta and delta cells.

- Alpha cells produce the hormone glucagon.
- Beta cells produce the hormone insulin.
- Delta cells produce the hormone somatostatin.

The two hormones insulin and glucagon have opposing effects.

Glucagon

This is a protein hormone that is released when the blood-glucose level drops too low. This happens in fasting or if there has been vomiting, or after exertion.

Glucagon has an action on:

- muscle cells, causing them to break down their stored glycogen and release glucose into the bloodstream.
- liver cells, causing them to break down their stored glycogen and release glucose into the bloodstream.
- liver and kidneys cells, stimulating them to produce glucose from fats and protein by gluconeogenesis and release it into the bloodstream.

Whenever you are not eating, that is when you are between meals or when you are sleeping, your body perceives it is starving. As a result the pancreas is stimulated to produce glucagon, to raise the blood-glucose so that the cells can be supplied with glucose.

Insulin

This is a protein hormone made up of 51 amino acids. It is the main hormone that regulates blood-glucose. When it is released into the blood stream it will exert an effect on all cells, but mainly upon the liver, fat cells and muscle cells.

Insulin has the opposite effect of glucagon. Insulin:

- stimulates all cells to take up glucose from the bloodstream.
- stimulates muscle cells to build and store glycogen.

- stimulates liver cells to build and store glycogen.
- stimulates liver and muscle cells to make protein from amino acids.
- stimulates fat cells to build and store fats from fatty acids and glycerol.
- inhibits liver and kidney cells from making further glucose from fatty acids or amino acids.

Thus when you eat, insulin is secreted. Its release is partly a result of the action of the vagus nerve, which is the tenth cranial nerve, and partly by stimulation of receptors that are triggered by glucose levels.

The action of insulin is to reduce the blood-glucose level to its comfortable level. It does this by stimulating the various reactions outlined above in the various organs. The net effect is to reduce the levels of glucose, fatty acids and amino acids in the blood and to cause nutrients to be stored in the organs and in fat.

Insulin is essentially a good housekeeper: it keeps your system tidy; maintains the level of glucose, amino acids and fatty acids in the blood at a safe level; and tucks energy-rich compounds, like glycogen protein and fats in their appropriate places.

If there is an excess of nutrients in the diet, then the storage may become apparent by the fat stores on the body getting larger and the person puts on weight.

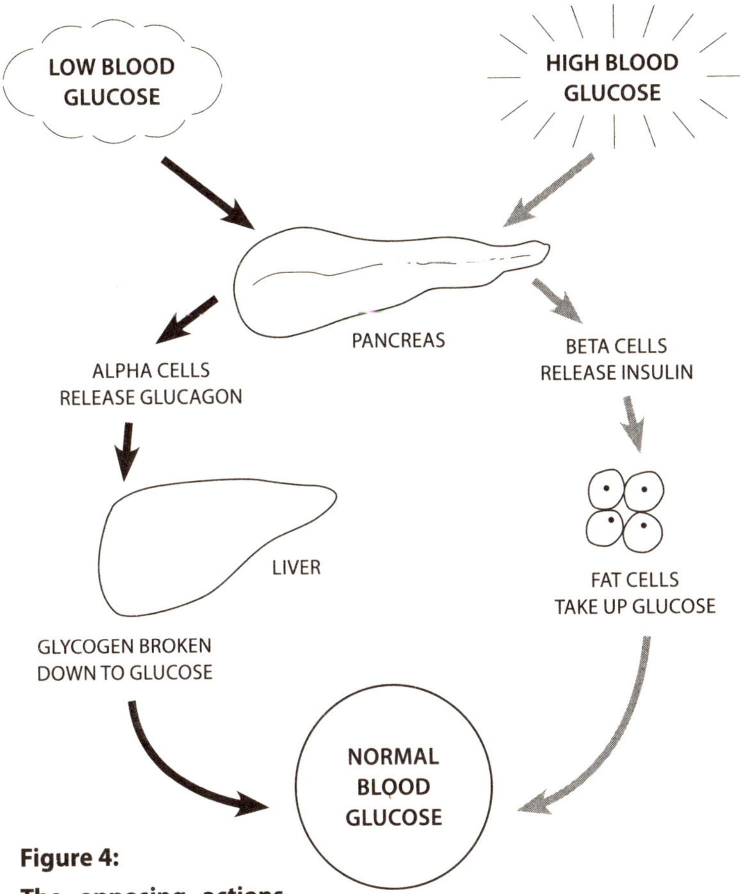

Figure 4:
The opposing actions of insulin and glucagon

We can see the opposing actions of insulin and glucagon in Figure 4.

Somatostatin

This hormone is produced in the delta cells in the islets of Langerhans in the pancreas and inhibits the secretion of other pancreatic hormones such as insulin and glucagon. Somatostatin is also produced in the gastrointestinal tract where it acts locally to reduce gastric secretion and the movements of the gastrointestinal tract. This helps to regulate the rate that food is absorbed from the contents inside the intestine.

The incretins, two lesser-known hormones

There are two other hormones that we need to consider. These have a part to play in regulating both insulin and glucagon. There are two of them:

- glucagon-like peptide 1 (GLP-1).
- glucose-dependent insulinotropic polypeptide (GIP).

They are both produced from small glands within the small intestine and their purpose is to:

- stimulate the production of insulin after you eat.
- reduce the production of glucagon by the liver during digestion, when it is not needed.
- slow digestion.
- decrease appetite.

That is all you need to know about these two hormones at this point. They have become of some importance in the treatment of Type 2 diabetes when control proves difficult with the first line drugs. We shall consider them in Chapter 9 (*Drugs for Type 2 diabetes*).

So what happens in diabetes?

We are now in a position to consider what happens in diabetes.

In Chapter 1, I mentioned that there are two main types of diabetes. In both types the lack of effective insulin action causes the blood-glucose to rise because of the following chain reaction.

1. The cells in the tissues cannot take up glucose.
2. With no glucose being absorbed by the cells, the body thinks it is starving and glucagon is released.
3. Glucagon stimulates breakdown of glycogen to release glucose into the blood.
4. Glucagon stimulates gluconeogenesis in the kidneys and the liver to release glucose into the blood.

The increased blood-glucose will result in glucose appearing in the urine. This is the main sign of diabetes and is, of course, why the condition was called diabetes mellitus, as we considered in Chapter 2 (*'The honey-sweet siphon' – the history of diabetes*).

This raised blood-glucose will also result in the symptoms of diabetes, which we looked at fleetingly in Chapter 1 (*An overview of diabetes*). We will look at the symptoms in more detail in Chapter 4 (*The symptoms of diabetes and how they come about*).

Chapter 4

The symptoms of diabetes and how they come about

In this chapter we are going to look at the classic symptoms of diabetes and the reasons why they occur. Many of these symptoms occur in Type 1 diabetes. Then we will look at other ways that diabetes may present, since Type 2 diabetes often smoulders on for a long time before it is recognised and diagnosed.

KEY POINTS

- Type 2 diabetes is often present five years before it is diagnosed.
- Diabetic complications affecting the eyes, kidneys, nerves and cardiovascular system are often present at the time of diagnosis.

The classic symptoms of diabetes are:

- thirst

- dehydration
- increased urinary frequency (polyuria)
- weight loss
- tiredness
- blurred vision
- increased susceptibility to infections.

You may wonder why raised blood-glucose is such a problem? Well, it is because of the strain that it throws on the body's metabolism and fluid balance.

Increased thirst and hunger

Both increased thirst and increased hunger can be quite marked.

Excessive thirst

Increased thirst, which is called polydipsia, can be throughout the whole day (even waking the person from sleep to have a drink) and the person can find that he or she craves fluids more than usual. The person may want to carry water round with him or her, when he or she did not have to beforehand, and have to replenish the bottle several times a day. It is also usually accompanied by a dry mouth, which has to be continually moistened.

KEY POINT

A thirst that cannot be quenched, in that you feel thirsty even after drinking, is suggestive of diabetes mellitus and has to be investigated.

The increased thirst comes about through several mechanisms.

- The blood-glucose directly stimulates thirst receptors in the brain, which make you want to drink.
- Increased urine flow results in loss of sodium. This again stimulates thirst receptors in the brain.

Increased hunger

Increased hunger, which is called polyphagia or hyperphagia can also occur, but may not be obvious to the person. Hunger, after all, does not seem as noticeable as increased thirst. Many people have what is often described as a healthy appetite; what is usually meant is that the person has a big appetite. It may not, of course, be healthy at all.

An increased hunger comes about because:

- a combination of lack of insulin and an increase in glucagon stimulates hunger receptors in the brain.
- cells deprived of glucose send out signals that the brain perceives to mean that the body is being starved. It stimulates hunger.
- increased thirst is often misperceived as increase in hunger.

Figure 5: Thirst and hunger mechanisms in diabetes

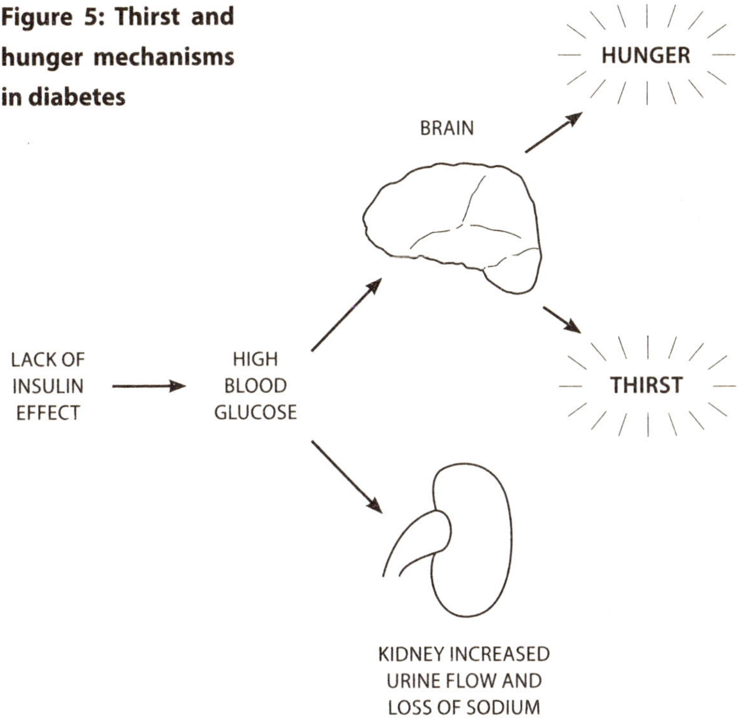

Increased frequency of urine

Polyuria is the name given for increased urinary frequency. It is caused by the effect of the raised blood-glucose on the kidneys.

The effect on the kidneys

To understand this we must consider the normal function of the kidneys.

There are two kidneys inside the abdomen. They are large bean-shaped organs, each about the size of the human fist. They are positioned below the ribcage on the back wall of the abdominal cavity. The right one is slightly lower than the left, because the right side of the abdomen has to accommodate the liver.

The main functions of the kidneys is to:

- filter the blood and remove waste products.
- prevent build up of fluid in the body.
- maintain levels of electrolytes, such as sodium, potassium and phosphate.
- produce hormones that:
    1. regulate blood pressure
    2. make red blood cells
    3. keep bones strong by maintaining calcium levels in the body.

The kidneys are effectively the body's great filtering organs. They filter the blood plasma, which is the blood's liquid. The kidneys maintain water balance and mineral and electrolyte balance and they pass waste product to the bladder in the urine.

In a healthy adult, the kidneys process around 200 litres of blood and produce around one to two litres of urine a day.

Each kidney is supplied with blood by a renal artery and drained by the renal vein. Each artery breaks up into a series of branches and is accompanied by a branch of the corresponding renal vein.

The filtering tissue is made up of microscopic filters called nephrons. Each kidney has about a million nephrons. These are contained in the renal medulla Thus you have about two million nephrons in the pair of kidneys.

The anatomy of the kidneys is shown in Figure 6 and the internal structure in Figure 6a.

Figure 6: The anatomical position of the kidneys inside the abdomen

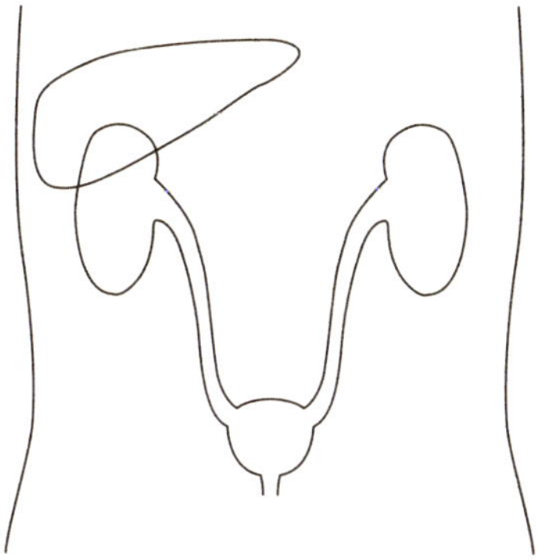

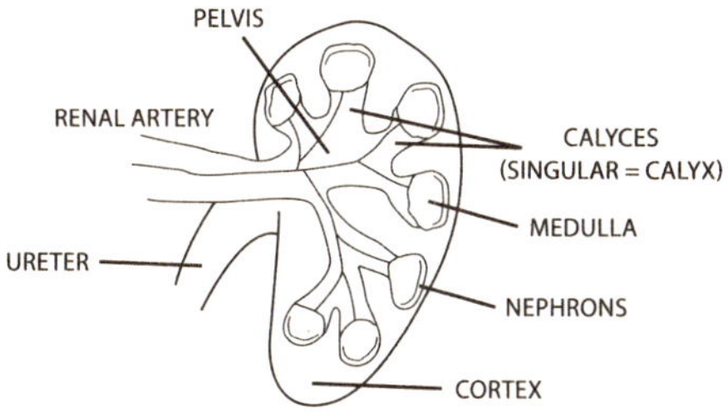

Figure 6a: Section through a kidney to show the internal structures of a kidney

The nephron is the actual filter unit. It consists of two main parts: the glomerulus and the tubule.

The glomerulus is a tiny spherical network of capillaries. It is surrounded by a structure called Bowman's capsule, which is connected to the tubule. Blood is supplied by an afferent arteriole. An arteriole is the very smallest type of artery, or blood vessel, that carries blood from the heart to the tissues. Afferent means it is the vessel going to a structure, in this case the arteriole feeding into the glomerulus.

The blood is drained out of the glomerulus by an efferent arteriole. This means that it is still a tiny artery carrying oxygen-rich blood from the heart, but efferent means that it is taking blood away from a structure, in this case away from the glomerulus. It continues on to supply the tubule.

The tubule is then drained by a tiny venule, which in turn drains into a vein. The vein carries blood back to the heart.

The nephron works in a two-step process.

- It lets fluid (plasma) and waste products pass through it, but it prevents cells and large molecules like proteins from passing through, leaving them in the bloodstream.
- The filtered fluid passes into the tubule, which removes waste and pumps needed minerals and electrolytes (such as sodium, potassium and phosphates) back to the bloodstream.

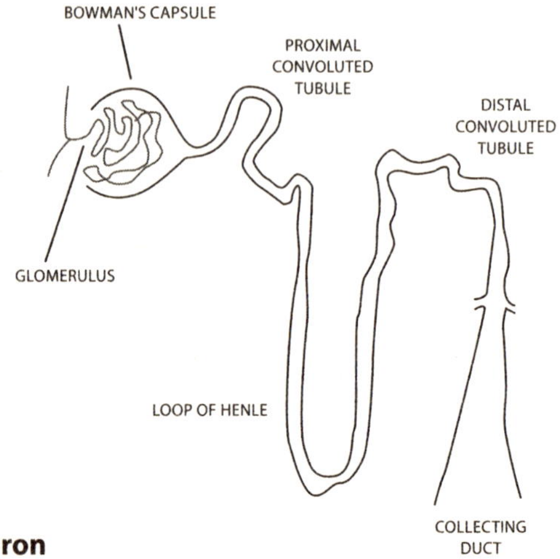

Figure 7: The nephron

In normal health the tubule is able to reabsorb all of the glucose from the filtered blood; normal fluid balance is thus maintained.

In diabetes there is increased frequency of urine because:

- blood-glucose is filtered through the glomerulus, but is too much for the tubule to manage.
- glucose is therefore left in the tubule.
- the glucose in the tubule causes water to be retained in the tubule causing increased urine flow to the bladder.
- more urine stretches the bladder and results in increased frequency of passage of urine.

Glycosuria is the name given to the presence of glucose in the urine. It is the cardinal sign of diabetes.

KEY POINT

The three Ps are the main symptoms of diabetes:

- polydipsia – increased thirst
- polyphagia – increased hunger
- polyuria – increased frequency of urination.

Dehydration

This comes about if the fluid loss exceeds the fluid intake. Dehydration can be worsened by:

- hot weather, resulting in increased fluid loss in perspiration.

- vomiting with increased fluid loss.
- diarrhoea with increased fluid loss.
- strenuous exercise.
- alcohol intake, because alcohol has a diuretic (fluid-losing) effect.

Weight change

Especially in Type 1 diabetes there may be weight loss. This comes about because:

- lack of insulin effect prevents glucose being transferred from the bloodstream into the cells.
- tissues try to generate fuel by burning fat in fat cells.
- tissues try to generate fuel by burning protein in muscle cells.

The result is a reduction in adipose (fat) tissue and muscle bulk.

Some people with Type 2 diabetes may experience this weight loss, but more often they experience weight gain. In fact, it may be the weight gain that causes the problem of Type 2 diabetes for many people. There is a definite increased risk of Type 2 diabetes with increasing excess weight. The reason may be that adipose or fat tissue is biochemically active and may induce insulin resistance.

Tiredness

This is essentially because the cells cannot absorb glucose. Glucose is the body's main fuel, so the cells have nothing to burn in order to produce energy. This may seem paradoxical, since the bloodstream is full of glucose. Yet the problem is that it cannot be used in the blood, it has to be metabolised through the Krebs cycle and the other pathways we looked at in Chapter 3 (*Metabolism and what goes wrong in diabetes*).

Blurred vision

The lenses of the eyes are subject to the same fluctuations in fluid balance as other bodily tissues. When the blood-glucose level rises, fluid is retained in the lens. This alters its focal length, causing an alteration in the way light is focused onto the retina within each eye. The effect is to produce blurring of the vision. It is correctible if the blood-glucose is controlled.

There are other possible causes of blurred vision in diabetes, which relate to complications caused by uncontrolled blood-glucose over a long time. We will discuss these in Chapter 7 (*The complications of diabetes*).

Increased susceptibility to infections

Diabetics are prone to infections. This heightened susceptibility can be due to several mechanisms.

- High blood-glucose levels impair the body's immune system, so infecting microbes can reproduce unchecked, resulting in the spread of an infection.
- Reduced blood flow to parts of the body as a result of the narrowing of blood vessels due to hardening of the arteries. This is called arteriosclerosis. We will look at it more closely in Chapter 5 (*The reasons why complications occur*).

- Damage to nerves, another recognised complication of diabetes, can result in reduced sensitivity of parts of the body. This is most likely to occur on the feet, as a diabetic neuropathy. Foot injuries can go unnoticed and an infection can get a hold. Again, we will consider this in more detail in Chapter 7 (*The complications of diabetes*).

Recurrent infections are common in diabetes. Indeed, they may be the reason for suspecting diabetes mellitus to be present. In particular the following infections are noted:

- fungal infections in skin creases, under the breasts, in armpits or around the groin
- vulval infections in women
- vaginal discharges (usually thrush)
- balanitis in men – an inflammation of the head of the penis or under the foreskin
- repeated athlete's foot
- repeated urinary infections
- repeated mouth infections, especially oral thrush
- increased itching of the skin.

Diabetes does not cause these infections, but it makes the person more susceptible to them and they can be harder to treat. In addition, other skin conditions such as psoriasis and acanthosis nigricans can result in damaged skin, which can become infected. See Chapter 7 (*The complications of diabetes*).

Slow healing of cuts and wounds

Cuts and scratches may seem to take longer to heal than they used to. This comes about if the small blood vessels are damaged by hardening of the arteries (arteriosclerosis). The body's natural healing process then becomes impaired.

Sometimes cuts and wounds may seem to fester. This can be the result of infection following the entry of microbes into the wound and reduction in the body's ability to clear the infection. This is the result of impairment of the immune process as mentioned in the last section on susceptibility to infection.

There may be no symptoms

This is very important, because many people with Type 2 diabetes have no symptoms at all or are not particularly bothered by them. They may not know that they have diabetes until they have a blood-glucose test done during routine examination at their doctor's surgery. This may, of course, initiate the other tests needed to confirm the diagnosis. We will consider this in Chapter 6 (*How diabetes is diagnosed and managed*).

The trouble is that there may be several years of raised blood-glucose levels, which may have been gradually damaging the body's various systems. Indeed, up to half of all people diagnosed with Type 2 diabetes will have complications at the time of diagnosis. In these cases, the symptoms that are the result of complications of diabetes can be the reason that someone consults their doctor.

Common symptoms of complications of diabetes include:

- in men, erectile difficulty. This can be difficulty in achieving or difficulty in maintaining an erection. It can be the result of both cardiovascular (arteriosclerosis or hardening of the arteries) complications and neurological (nerve) complications.
- numbness or weakness in the extremities.
- tingling in the hands, feet or legs. This may be the result of neuropathy (nerve damage).
- visual disturbances, including loss of some of the visual field or even blindness.
- an ulcer on a foot or leg.
- coldness of the feet, from arteriosclerosis.
- gangrenous changes in the toes.
- chest pain on exertion. This can be from angina, because of arteriosclerosis of the coronary arteries, which supply the heart.
- shortness of breath on exertion, which may indicate cardiovascular problems with the heart.

KEY POINTS

- Many people have diabetes for five years before it is diagnosed.
- Diabetes UK estimate that up to 850,000 adults in the UK have diabetes but are not aware of it.
- Fifty per cent of newly diagnosed Type 2 diabetics will already have cardiovascular disease.

Chapter 5

The reasons why complications occur

This chapter focuses on the underlying mechanisms that result in diabetes complications. In medicine this means looking a little at the pathology, or the science of disease.

KEY POINTS

- Complications of diabetes may never occur.
- Good control of the diabetes can prevent them from occurring.

The causes of the complications

Diabetes can affect virtually any part of the body and any of its organ systems. We are not entirely sure how the complications arise, but it seems probable that the following four mechanisms are involved.

1. The arterial system, to cause arteriosclerosis or hardening of the arteries.
2. Excessive amounts of chemicals called advanced glycation end products (or AGEs) impair the function of various cells and tissues.
3. Excessive glucose overloads the glycolysis pathway (see Chapter 3: *Metabolism and what goes wrong in diabetes*) so another metabolic pathway is used resulting in the production of sorbitol. This is a polyol that accumulates in tissues and seems to damage the cells directly, causing them to swell and lose their functioning ability.
4. The nervous system, which sends nerves to all parts of the body. If the nerves that control organs are damaged then the organs may not function correctly.

Before we look at the individual complications we will look at these four processes as they can give us a greater understanding of how damage occurs.

1. Hardening of the arteries

The medical name for hardening of the arteries is arteriosclerosis. It is a normal part of ageing as the pressure inside makes the vessel walls harder and stiffer. It is accelerated as a complication of diabetes.

Arteriosclerosis and atherosclerosis

These two terms are often used interchangeably. Atherosclerosis is actually a specific type of arteriosclerosis that causes the macro-vascular complications of diabetes. Macro-vascular means affecting the large arteries. Thus:

- coronary heart disease – affecting the blood supply of the heart.
- cerebrovascular disease – affecting the blood supply of the brain.
- peripheral vascular disease – affecting the blood supply of the limbs.

Atherosclerosis comes from the Latinised version of the Greek, *athero*, meaning gruel or porridge, and the Greek *sclerosis*, meaning hardening. This image then of producing a hardened porridge-like interior to the artery walls is not far from what happens. The lining of the blood vessels accumulates a patchy covering that is fatty, grainy, rough and sticky, like gruel or porridge.

KEY POINT

There are three factors that can all contribute to the damage to the blood vessels:

- raised blood-glucose
- raised cholesterol and other blood fat levels
- raised blood pressure.

All of these may be involved in the pathological process of arteriosclerosis, or hardening of the arteries.

KEY POINTS

- Atherosclerosis is the basic problem that causes coronary artery disease, cerebrovascular disease and peripheral vascular disease.
- Atherosclerosis is the process in which atheroma is laid down in arteries.

- Atheroma (the 'gruel' that accumulates inside the artery lining) may restrict blood flow.
- Rupture of an atheroma plaque can cause a clot to form inside a blood vessel.

The anatomical structure of the arteries

If we look at a cross section through an artery we can delineate three layers.

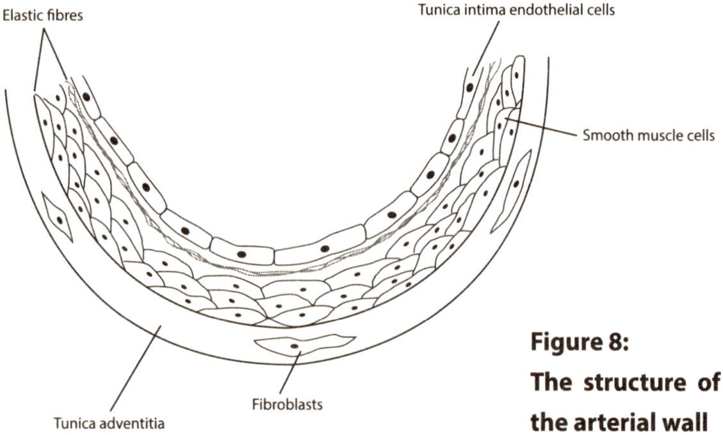

Figure 8: The structure of the arterial wall

Tunica intima – this is the innermost layer, and it consists of flat cells that are arranged rather like paving stones to produce a smooth surface. The cells are called endothelial cells. They are stuck together by a glue of polysaccharides (long carbohydrate molecules made up of repeating units of sugars). Underneath, they have a connective tissue coating of elastic tissue called the internal elastic lamina.

Tunica media – this is the middle and thickest layer of artery walls. It is essentially elastic connective tissue and smooth muscle cells. It is surrounded by another layer of elastic tissue called the external elastic lamina.

Tunica adventitia – this is connective tissue that contains nerves and tiny capillaries, which supply the cells of the vessel.

The space inside the blood vessel, through which blood flows, is called the lumen.

The pathological process – what actually happens

The process of the hardening of the arteries is a slow, gradual build up over many years. It goes on without the individual being aware of any problem, until the blood flow is so reduced that symptoms appear when the heart is called upon to pump more blood, or if a clot and a sudden blockage of the artery in question occurs.

In diabetes the arterial walls are damaged by three factors:

Blood-glucose

Over years the blood-glucose causes the inner lining of the blood vessel to absorb more glucose than usual. This results in the lining becoming thicker and weaker.

Cholesterol

Cholesterol is a fat, which tends to increase in diabetics. The raised level that results in the blood can become laid down in blood vessels, as we shall see in the section below – How the atheroma fatty plaques build up – and illustrated in Figure 9.

High blood pressure

The longer the blood pressure is raised, the greater is the risk of damage to blood vessels. It can affect all sizes of arteries, from the very smallest arterioles, to the medium sized coronary arteries and even the large aorta.

When damage occurs to the lining of an arterial blood vessel, atheroma plaques, also called fatty plaques, develop inside the vessel wall, which will have an effect not unlike the silting up of a riverbed. As a result, blood flow to the tissues supplied is reduced. These plaques can encircle the whole lining of the artery or may be quite eccentric and just a bleb (rounded growth) on a part of the internal artery wall.

How the atheroma fatty plaques build up

The plaque is the result of a process that starts when endothelial cells get damaged. When this happens, there is a reduction in the production of various defensive chemicals and hormones, whose role it is to maintain the integrity of the cells.

Circulating white blood cells (leucocytes) are attracted to the damaged area and bind to the endothelial cells. Then they migrate through the endothelial lining to lie underneath it. They tend to become transformed into macrophages, which are large cells whose function is to engulf and digest debris and microbial invaders. The name comes from the Greek *makros,* meaning big, and *phagein,* meaning eat. They are 'big eaters.' What they then do is scavenge and absorb LDL cholesterol (the bad cholesterol) and become foam cells. These are characteristic of atheroma plaques.

The earliest lesions are called fatty streaks and they simply consist of these foam cells. Gradually they absorb calcium and they develop a fibrous coating, as smooth muscle cells get transformed into fibre.

By this stage the atheroma is producing a lump that will start to intrude into the lumen of the artery.

The developing atheroma plaque gradually becomes more organised and develops a fibrous cap. The interior of the atheroma plaque consists of foam cells, cholesterol crystals and calcium. It really deserves the porridge-like description of atheroma. While this fibrous cap remains intact, blood flows over it and symptoms may not occur.

Lots of atheroma lesions can develop along the course of an artery, the net effect being to narrow it along a significant length, thereby reducing the flow of blood through it. If this happens in the coronary arteries, which supply the heart, then angina may be the result.

Atheroma is most likely to build up at curves in the arteries, or where branches and tributaries are thrown off from a main trunk.

All of this process has the effect of altering the structure of the artery wall, so that it becomes much less elastic, much more rigid and much more vulnerable; it becomes hardened.

It can take thirty years or more to develop significant atherosclerosis in someone without diabetes. By comparison, in someone with undiagnosed diabetes this can take a mere ten years.

The danger point is reached when an atheromatous plaque ulcerates, like a miniature volcano, to cause thrombus formation, possibly with a cataclysmic result. Such ruptures of plaques can occur from forty years of age and upwards.

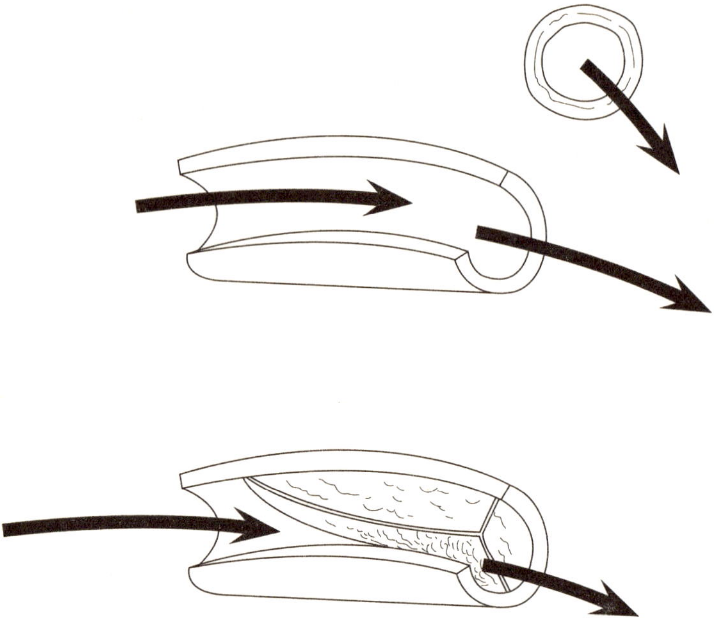

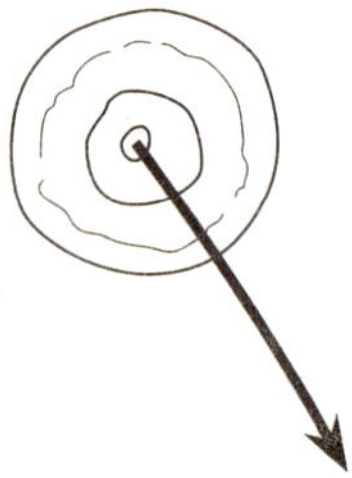

Figure 9:
The build up of atheroma
Top: Normal artery with unrestricted blood flow
Bottom: Diseased artery in which atheroma plaque restricts blood flow

Thrombosis

In atherosclerosis a plaque or atheroma can suddenly rupture and a cascade reaction occurs which produces a clot to form over the ruptured plaque in order to seal the damaged wall. It is essentially a normal body reaction to self-seal a damaged area. The unfortunate thing is that the cells that are being mobilised to do so, and which fulfil the function that they are designed for, have no awareness that they could be causing a clot to form that could be catastrophic for the whole organism.

An atheroma plaque can rupture if its pulp becomes necrotic, which means some of the cells inside it die, or if it just becomes too big to be contained by the fibrous capsule.

As long as the integrity of the epithelial lining is maintained, then the blood will flow. However, if that layer is disrupted by the rupture of a plaque, then messenger chemicals will alert blood cells, which will move to the area to form a clot to seal off the damaged part of the vessel. Platelets will accumulate and a fibrous structure resembling a spider's web will be formed to catch more cells to help to seal the damage. This is called a thrombus. The process of thrombus formation is called thrombosis.

Figure 10: Thrombosis or clot formation

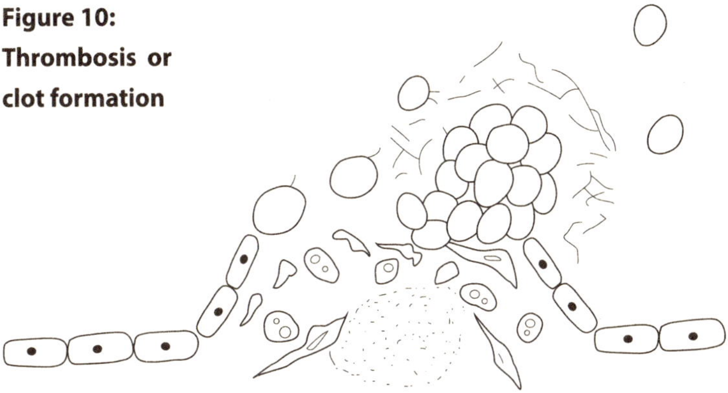

If a thrombus or clot forms in an already narrowed coronary artery (which supplies the heart muscle) and blocks off the flow of blood, then a heart attack is likely. The part of the heart that is supplied by that artery will die.

Similarly, if a cerebral artery (which supplies part of the brain) is blocked off, then it can cause a stroke.

The role of platelets

The platelets are the very smallest blood cells. They do not have any nucleus and they live for a mere ten days. They are continually produced and die off, so that there are a constant number of them. Their function is to plug and heal wounds by clumping together to form clots. They are therefore an integral part of the body's clotting mechanism.

Inside a tiny blood vessel, when a plaque ruptures, chemicals are leached into the circulation and then platelets and other blood cells in the vicinity move to the damaged area under the action of various natural chemicals, including prostaglandins. Then an enzyme in the platelets, called cyclo-oxygenase 1 is activated. This causes the platelets to stick together and accumulate in the fibrous web structure to produce the thrombus.

Blockage of arteries causes two problems

If an artery is only partially blocked, but allows a flow of blood to the tissues then it may not cause any symptoms. Symptoms may occur when a critical point is reached, or if the system is asked to do extra work necessitating more oxygen. The impaired circulation cannot provide this and the tissues become deprived of oxygen.

Ischaemia

The body's tissues all need oxygen for their functioning and survival. Whenever the blood supply is inadequate, the tissue is said to have become ischaemic. Different types of tissue have different oxygen needs. Connective tissue can survive better than epithelial tissue. Heart tissue and nerve tissue, especially brain cells, cannot survive more than a few seconds without oxygen. Similarly, the myocardium, the muscle of the heart, cannot sustain ischaemia for long. The consequence is pain.

Infarction

When deprived of oxygen beyond a critical point, cells start to die. This is called infarction. The infarction of heart muscle may lead to instant cardiac failure and sudden death. Myocardial infarction is the name we give to a heart attack. It means that some of the heart muscle (myocardium) has been damaged and dies.

2. Advanced glycation end products or AGEs

There is a great deal of research going on into substances called advanced glycation end products as a cause of complications in diabetes.[6] These were first discovered in 1912, but it has only been over the last three decades that their importance in health has been appreciated.

AGEs have been implicated in the development of a whole range of conditions including Alzheimer's disease, cancer, heart disease, high blood pressure, kidney disease and the general process of ageing.

They are essentially body proteins and lipids (fats), which are damaged by a process called glycation. This causes glucose to become attached to protein molecules to produce an advanced glycation end product, or AGE. These reduce or stop the function of the protein. Thus enzymes, which are made of proteins, can become ineffective, causing marked diminution of many metabolic processes in cells.

In normal circumstances, blood-glucose will become glycated to haemoglobin, the red pigment in red blood cells. This forms HbA1c, which is used as a marker of diabetic control as we shall see later. Similarly, albumin, a blood protein, can become glycated with glucose to form glycated albumin.

When there is excess blood-glucose, as in diabetes, then glucose can become glycated to all sorts of cells. In general this reduces their functioning. For example, HbA1c is 'stickier' than ordinary haemoglobin, so it holds onto its oxygen for longer and doesn't give it up to the tissues as well. The result is that the tissues do not receive as much oxygen as they need. White blood cells become less efficient and less able to fight infections, and infections are a problem for diabetics, of course.

The body can cope with a certain level of AGEs, but if it is too much, which will occur with prolonged excessively high blood-glucose, these AGEs can damage tissues in the eyes, the kidneys and the nerves.

3. The polyol pathway

In Chapter 3 (*Metabolism and what goes wrong in diabetes*), I described the glycolysis pathway as a metabolic route by which glucose is converted into pyruvate to free energy. In diabetes there is too much glucose for the glycolysis pathway to handle, so glucose is channelled into an alternative metabolic process called the polyol pathway.

Polyols are alcohols containing a hydroxyl group (a functional group in a molecule consisting of an atom of oxygen and an atom of hydrogen).

Glucose is reduced to sorbitol, a type of polyol, by the enzyme aldose reductase. Under normal circumstances the sorbitol is then oxidised to fructose, another sugar, by the enzyme sorbitol dehydrogenase. In diabetes, this gets overwhelmed and excess sorbitol is produced.

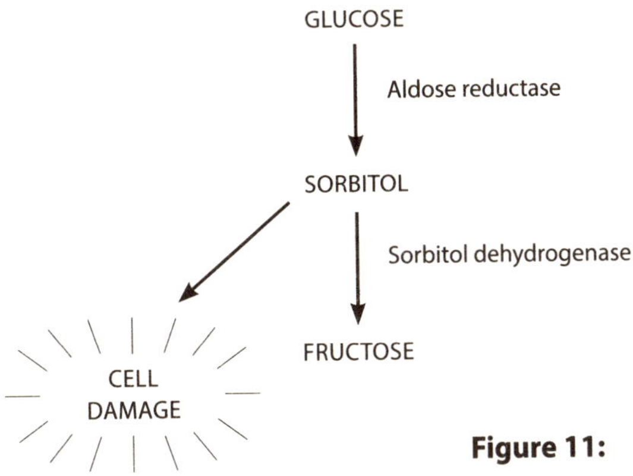

Figure 11:
The polyol pathway

The sorbitol accumulates in tissues and seems to damage the cells directly, by interfering with the metabolic processes, or by causing them to swell and lose their functioning ability.

4. Nerve damage

Neurones are the nerve cells. These are the basic functional cells of the nervous system. There are actually many different types of neurones, which come in different shapes and sizes depending on where they are situated in the nervous system and their function.

The basic structure of a neurone consists of a body (called a soma), an axon and dendrites. The axon carries information away from the body of the cell, otherwise known as the soma, whereas the dendrites, which are wispy, tentacle-like projections, receive information and convey it to the body.

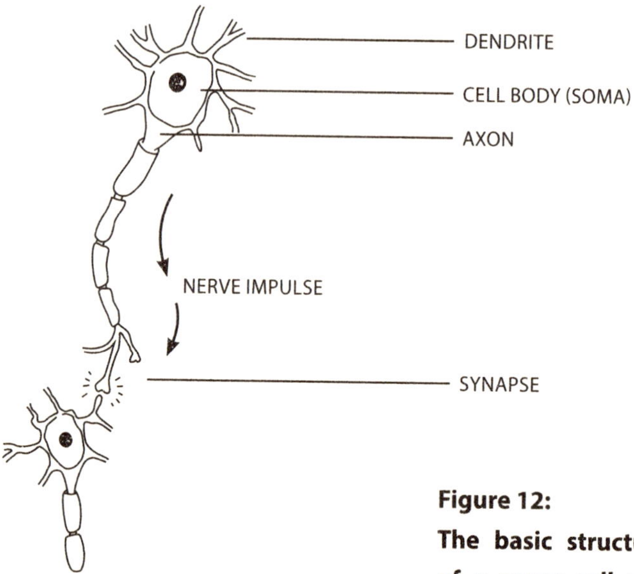

Figure 12:
The basic structure of a nerve cell and normal function

The axon is coated in a myelin sheath, which acts rather like the insulating coating of an electrical wire, to stop electrical impulses being discharged too early.

Damage to nerves in diabetes seems to come about through the combined effect of the three processes we have discussed. The hardening of arteries affects the micro-vessels supplying the nerves, so that they receive less blood supply than they need. Thus they get less oxygen, which is necessary for the cells to function.

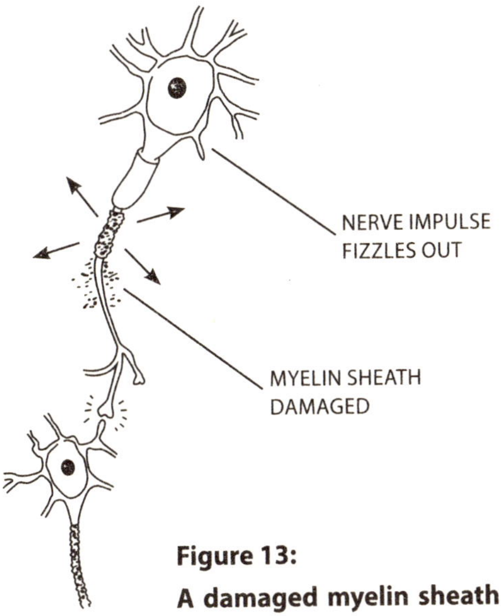

Figure 13:
A damaged myelin sheath allows a nerve impulse to fizzle out

The excess amount of AGEs and the sorbitol can directly damage the myelin sheaths. As a result the normal electrical impulse up or down a nerve is impaired and the nerve impulse effectively fizzles out and does not reach wherever it was meant to go. In the case of a motor nerve, one of the nerves that supply a muscle or organ, the impulse does not reach it from the brain so the part does not function. In the case of a sensory nerve, which carries sense impulses (touch, temperature sensation or pain sensation), the impulse will not reach the brain. Hence numbness or other sense impairment results.

Complications can affect many of the body's systems

Metabolic

These are generally problems with the sugar levels, either from the condition or its treatment. Metabolic problems tend to be acute or short-term complications, in that that they take place rapidly. Because they can happen rapidly, they can be dangerous so medical help is usually needed as an emergency.

Cardiovascular

These can be subdivided into:

1. Macro-vascular – these are complications arising from arteriosclerosis or hardening of the large blood arteries.

- Coronary arteries: supplying the heart to cause angina and heart attacks.
- Peripheral arteries: supplying the limbs to produce intermittent claudication, which is a painful cramp in the legs on walking.
- Cerebral arteries: supplying the brain to cause strokes.

2. Micro-vascular – these are complications arising from arteriosclerosis or hardening of the arterioles, the tiny blood vessels that supply the tissues.

- Blood vessels: in the retinae of the eyes to cause diabetic retinopathy.
- Blood vessels: in the kidneys to cause diabetic nephropathy.
- Blood vessels: in the tissues to cause ulceration and other problems.

Kidney and bladder problems

The kidney can be affected, resulting in chronic kidney disease and possible renal failure. Nerve control may be affected resulting in incontinence and increased frequency of urinary infections.

Neurological

This can result in problems with vision, pain or numbness or tingling in the extremities, or difficulties caused by nerve supply to organs.

Immune impairment

The reduction in the white cells' ability to attack and deal with invading organisms can be reduced by the AGEs effect outlined earlier, when glucose sticks to protein in their cell membranes. Also, the reduced blood supply to tissues impedes the body's ability to mount an adequate inflammatory response to repel and deal with invading bacteria.

Cataracts and other visual problems

The eyes can be affected as a result of hardening of the arteries, nerve damage and alteration in the lenses of the eyes.

Erectile dysfunction and loss of libido

This can be a huge issue, which we will consider in Chapter 10 (*Using the Life Cycle with Type 2 diabetes*).

Stomach and bowel problems

These can arise as a result of damage to the blood and nerve supply of the digestive tract.

Bladder problems

The bladder sensation may become reduced, leading to urine dribbling and incomplete bladder emptying, leading to an increased number of urinary infections.

Limb problems

These can be the result of peripheral artery disease (mentioned previously) and poor wound healing, which culminates in leg ulceration. This can be compounded by the increased susceptibility to infection that occurs in diabetes. In addition, other structural problems can affect the feet in diabetes.

Psychological problems

It is common for people to experience stress and anxiety, sleep difficulties and depression as a result of having diabetes.

Part Two

DEALING WITH TYPE 2 DIABETES

Looking after your diabetes is a partnership between yourself and the health professionals. It is important to appreciate that you have a large part to play in actively managing the diabetes. It is not simply a matter of taking medication to keep the blood-glucose and more particularly the HbA1c under control.

Blood-sugar levels are like taking a snapshot of the state of your diabetes, whereas HbA1c is like taking a video. It gives you an idea of how the diabetes has been controlled over the preceding two or three months.

Chapter 6

How diabetes is diagnosed and managed

From Part 1 you will have seen that it is important to diagnose diabetes as early in the process as possible, in order to gain good control of blood-glucose and prevent complications.

Type 2 diabetes is usually diagnosed by the GP either at a routine examination or when the person consults after having noticed some of the symptoms of diabetes. (See Chapter 4: *The symptoms of diabetes and how they come about*.)

Sometimes it is because of a complication of diabetes, such as persistent and irritant thrush in the vagina in women or under the foreskin in men or oral thrush in both sexes.

Sometimes people take advantage of having a blood test done at a pharmacist or as part of an assessment at a sports or leisure club, and are then referred to the GP.

Still others may be referred by their optician, who may have noticed signs of retinopathy on examination of their retinae at an eye examination.

Diabetes UK estimates that there are around 850,000 people in England with undiagnosed diabetes.

DIFFERENT UNITS OF MEASUREMENT

Blood-glucose measurements

In the UK blood-glucose is generally measured in mmol/l (millimoles per litre).

In Europe and the USA blood-glucose is measured in mg/dl (milligrams per decilitre, where a decilitre is a tenth of a litre or 100 millilitres). Both sets of units are used to measure blood-sugar levels and both give a measurement of the concentration of glucose in the blood, albeit in slightly different ways.

- The unit mmol/l gives the molarity, which is the number of molecules of a substance within a specified volume, in this case within one litre.
- The unit mg/dl gives the concentration by the ratio of weight to volume, in this case, milligrams per decilitre.

If you use a glucose meter then you can usually convert from one to the other.

HbA1c measurements

This test used to be measured as a percentage of the haemoglobin affected. Now it is measured in mmol/mol. Note the difference between blood-glucose measured in mmol/l and HbA1c, measured in mmol/mol.

The initial tests

The GP is likely to do two tests with a urine test first as it is non-invasive. In normal health (as explained in Chapter 4: *The symptoms of diabetes and how they come about*) glucose does not appear in the urine. The presence of glucose in the urine, called glycosuria, is significant. It does not always mean that diabetes is present, since sometimes there can be a lowering of the threshold at which glucose is excreted by the kidneys such as in pregnancy (although even then it has to be checked to exclude gestational diabetes).

The sample of urine is tested with a test strip that changes colour in the presence of glucose. The higher the glucose level, the greater the colour change. This sample may also be sent off to the laboratory for urinalysis and microscopic examination and culturing to see whether there is any infection present.

After a positive urine test a finger prick test involves pricking the end of a finger with a small gadget that produces a few drops of blood. These are then applied to a test strip, which is put into a small glucose meter. This will then give a reading of the blood-glucose.

If the GP considers it necessary, then a larger blood sample may be taken and sent off to the hospital laboratory for accurate testing of the blood-glucose.

The following are tests used to diagnose diabetes.

Random blood-glucose

A random blood-glucose taken at any time, is usually done to check for Type 1 diabetes. If it shows a level above 11.0 mmol/l (millimoles per litre) it is diagnostic of diabetes.

A random blood-glucose of less that 11.0 mmol/l does not, on the other hand, mean that no diabetes is present. If it had been taken after food then it could have been pushed up to 10.5, for example, but could later drop below the diagnostic level. If it was a sample several hours after food then it may be significant and would need further clarification with one of the below tests.

Fasting blood-glucose

This is a blood sample taken in the morning before eating, after an overnight fast, so that there have been eight to ten hours since the last meal. It can diagnose diabetes or pre-diabetes.

- A level of 7.0 mmol/l is diagnostic of diabetes if the person has symptoms of diabetes. If they do not have symptoms of diabetes, yet have a level above 7.0 mmol/l the test needs to be repeated.
- A level between 6.1 and 6.9 mmol/l is impaired fasting glucose or pre-diabetes.
- A level below 6.0 mmol/l is normal.

Oral glucose tolerance test

If the diagnosis is still in doubt, then an oral glucose tolerance test (or OGTT) will be ordered. This is again done as a fasting test, after an eight- to ten-hour fast. A fasting sample is taken in the morning then the person is given a drink containing 75 grams of glucose. A blood sample is taken two hours later. If diabetes is not present the body handles this glucose load and after two hours the level will drop.

There are three ranges that are given in the OGTT with both the fasting level and the two hours after the glucose load level.

1. Fasting test level:

- above 7.0 mmol/l – diagnostic of diabetes.
- 6.0–7.0 mmol/l – impaired glucose tolerance or pre-diabetes.
- less than 6.0 mmol/l – normal.

2. Two hours after glucose load level:

- 11.1 mmol/l or above – diagnostic of diabetes.
- 7.8–11.1 mmol/l – impaired glucose tolerance or pre-diabetes.
- less than 7.8 mmol/l – normal, non-diabetic level.

Once Type 2 diabetes is diagnosed, the person will be regularly followed-up by the GP and the practice nurse, with input from other professionals like podiatrists and dieticians.

A normal result needs no further investigation, but anything within the impaired glucose tolerance or pre-diabetes range is important, as we shall consider in the sections below.

The glycated haemoglobin or HbA1c test

As I mentioned in Chapter 5: The reasons why complications occur, blood-glucose will stick to the haemoglobin, the red pigment that carries oxygen in red blood cells. This stickiness is called glycation and the glycated haemoglobin is called HbA1c.

This has been the standard means of monitoring diabetes for many years.

It is nowadays increasingly used to diagnose Type 2 diabetes or pre-diabetes, as advised by the World Health Organization (WHO) in 2011. The reason it has been chosen is because Type 2 diabetes and pre-diabetes usually do not just suddenly occur, but build up gradually without the person being aware. That means that the blood-glucose will have been high for a long time. The HbA1c is effectively a measure of the blood-glucose over the previous two to three months. It has the advantage over the other tests in that it can be carried out at any time of the day, since it is not going to fluctuate whereas the blood-glucose does. It also does not require any fasting.

The WHO suggests the following diagnostic guidelines for diabetes:

- HbA1c below 42.0 mmol/mol (6.0 per cent) – non-diabetic.
- HbA1c between 42.0 and 47.0 mmol/mol (6.0–6.4 per cent) – impaired glucose regulation or pre-diabetes.
- HbA1c of 48 mmol/mol (6.5 per cent) or over – Type 2 diabetes.

Prior to 2011 the HbA1c was measured as a percentage of the haemoglobin affected, so many patients and doctors were used to measuring it as a percentage figure. In line with international recording, it is now recorded in mmol/mol.

Pre-diabetes

Pre-diabetes, which is also commonly called borderline diabetes, is a stage in which the blood-glucose is persistently raised, but not high enough to be diagnosed as diabetes.

It is sometimes referred to as impaired glucose tolerance, which means that the individual is not able to tolerate a high glucose load, or at least, not able to handle it as well as someone without diabetes.

It is an important stage, because diabetes can be prevented. In the UK it is estimated that there are currently about seven million people with pre-diabetes. All of them, by implication are at risk of developing diabetes.

Research has actually also shown that the prevalence of pre-diabetes has been going steadily upwards between 2003 and 2011, so that 35.5 per cent of the adult population in England has pre-diabetes.[7] That is more than one adult in every three who is at risk of eventually developing diabetes.

KEY POINT

According to the WHO, a healthy diet, regular physical activity, maintaining a normal body weight and avoiding tobacco use can prevent or delay the onset of Type 2 diabetes.

How do I know if I have pre-diabetes?

Pre-diabetes may produce no symptoms whatsoever. That will probably come as no surprise to you if you have read the book so far, since many people actually have diabetes for several years before it is diagnosed. During that time the persistently raised blood-glucose may have been having some damaging effect on the blood vessels and the nerves.

An individual with pre-diabetes may only become aware of the diagnosis after blood testing. The blood testing may be a routine examination at the doctor's surgery or it may be after the development of one or other of the early signs of diabetes.

Risk factors for pre-diabetes and Type 2 diabetes

The following factors increase the risk of developing both pre-diabetes and Type 2 diabetes:

- being overweight or obese.

- having a waist measurement of more than 80 centimetres for women, or 94 centimetres for men.
- having a strong family history of diabetes – a parent or a sibling.
- increasing age over 40 years.
- ethnicity – higher risk in Hispanic people, Native Americans, Asians and Africans.
- hypertension.
- on lipid testing, having a low HDL, or 'good', cholesterol level or having a high triglyceride level.
- women having had a large baby over the weight of four kilograms.
- inactive lifestyle – if the person does less than 30 minutes of physical activity a day.
- if diet is devoid of fruit and vegetables.

INCREASED RISK OF CANCER

Research analysing 16 studies that included almost 999,000 people from around the world with pre-diabetes found that people with pre-diabetes had a 15 per cent increased risk of cancer.[8]

Differentiating between pre-diabetes and Type 2 diabetes

The important thing to appreciate is that having pre-diabetes gives you an opportunity to prevent it becoming diabetes. Left to its own devices, without any change in lifestyle, pre-diabetes will become diabetes. This can take up to ten years, but it could be less than one year.

The differentiation between pre-diabetes and diabetes is entirely dependent on the levels of the HbA1c.

- HbA1c below 42.0 mmol/mol (6.0 per cent) – non-diabetic.
- HbA1c between 42.0 and 47.0 mmol/mol (6.0–6.4 per cent) – impaired glucose regulation or pre-diabetes.
- HbA1c of 48.0 mmol/mol (6.5 per cent or over) – Type 2 diabetes.

People at risk of pre-diabetes or Type 2 diabetes, in the above list, should be tested once every three years. Once pre-diabetes has developed, the test should be every year.

METABOLIC SYNDROME

This is a combination of risk factors, which are known to increase the risk of heart disease, stroke and Type 2 diabetes.

According to the International Diabetes Federation (IDF):

- 25 per cent of the world's adult population have metabolic syndrome.
- people with metabolic syndrome are three times as likely to have a heart attack or stroke as people without it.
- people with metabolic syndrome are five times as likely to develop diabetes as people without it.
- a metabolic syndrome is diagnosed if:
    - waist circumference is 101 centimetres or more for men and 89 centimetres or more for women.
    - raised triglycerides level.

- reduced HDL ('good') cholesterol.
- elevated blood pressure (130/85 mm Hg or higher).
- elevated fasting glucose.

Preventing Type 2 diabetes

This is a very important section, so if you find that you fall into the pre-diabetes range I cannot emphasise enough, do not be complacent. Do your utmost to prevent Type 2 diabetes, since by doing so you reduce your risk of developing complications of diabetes.

Avoid obesity and get your weight down

It is known that increasing levels of obesity are associated with increased incidence of Type 2 diabetes and heart disease.

The early death rate of people who are 13.5–18 kilograms overweight is 30 per cent greater than one would expect in a general population of people of normal weight. More alarmingly, there is a 50 per cent increase in early death for men who weigh more than 40 per cent above ideal body weight.

Ideally you should aim for a body mass index (BMI) of 18.5–25.0. Body mass index is an accepted means of relating weight to height. It is worked out by dividing the weight in kilograms by the square of the height in metres. You can find BMI calculators on the Internet and get an immediate result. It is essentially giving an estimation of human body fat, although it does not actually measure fat. You can also refer to Figure 19 in Chapter 8 (*Lifestyle changes to treat Type 2 diabetes*).

IT IS BETTER TO BE A PEAR THAN AN APPLE

You may have heard this one. It relates to the distribution of your excess body fat. Fat accumulated around the abdomen, the classic beer belly, has a high correlation with the risk of coronary heart disease and Type 2 diabetes.

This can be measured by comparing the ratio of the waist to the hips. A high waist to hips ratio (beer belly) will tend to make one look like an apple. By contrast, a slimmer abdomen and larger hips has a lower waist-hips ratio and a lower risk. The body is more pear-shaped.

Visceral fat, that is the fat that accumulates inside the abdomen and produces the beer-belly shape, is associated with insulin resistance. Indeed, research shows a strong correlation with Type 2 diabetes, so it really is better to be a pear than an apple.

Another measure of obesity that is perhaps more accurate than a BMI is the waist–height ratio. That is your waist measurement divided by your height. It should be less than 0.5 to give a low risk. Once it gets above half (0.5) then the risk is increased, and the greater the figure the greater the risk. It seems to be a better indicator because BMI makes no distinction between muscle and fat. The waist–height ratio, on the other hand is purely an indicator of your body proportions.

This was demonstrated by researchers at Oxford Brookes University in the UK[9] who examined data on patients whose BMI and waist to height ratio were measured in the 1980s. Twenty years later, death rates among the group were much more closely linked to participants' earlier waist to height ratio than their BMI, suggesting it is a more useful tool for identifying health risks at an early stage.

KEY POINT

As a rule of thumb, a waist circumference of more than 101 centimetres for men and 89 centimetres for women indicates a high risk of coronary artery disease.

Avoid inactivity

You need to exercise for at least 30 minutes a day, but as we will see in Chapter 8 (*Lifestyle changes to treat Type 2 diabetes*), this does not mean that you have to exercise vigorously. There are other strategies you can use.

For example, older people who are at risk may be interested to know that walking for just 15 minutes three times a day after meals is better for you than a single walk of 45 minutes once a day. Those short walks may seem more manageable and, when they are done after meals, they seem to control blood-glucose levels more effectively.

The study that supports this was carried out on older adults who were all classified as obese, with a body mass index of more than 30. Their average age was 70. Their 24-hour blood-glucose readings were measured when they had no exercise, when they had a 45-minute morning or evening walk and when they took three 15-minute walks half an hour after meals. All of the walks lowered the blood-glucose levels, but the short walks reduced it the most effectively.

The gap of half an hour after a meal was in order to allow for digestion. Within that 30 minutes, glucose floods into the blood. Then using the muscles starts to clear the glucose from the blood. Effectively, the muscles help the pancreas to clear the blood. If you do this regularly, the glucose goes to the muscles to help their metabolism. The result is reduction in blood-glucose, which helps lower the risk of diabetes. This would certainly seem to be a sensible thing for older adults who are overweight to incorporate into their lifestyle. It needs to become a daily thing, not just something that you do occasionally, in order to reap the benefits.

Increase your fibre intake

It has been shown in several studies that low fibre intake is associated with higher incidence of Type 2 diabetes. It has been clearly demonstrated that a higher intake of fibre reduces the risk of metabolic syndrome, which is itself a risk for Type 2 diabetes.[10] Further, a study of African-American women showed clearly that a diet high in fibre was associated with a lower risk of Type 2 diabetes.[11]

Drink coffee

This might surprise you. There has been a lot of interest in coffee consumption and the risk of developing Type 2 diabetes. Several meta-analyses have been undertaken, all of which indicate that a higher consumption of coffee is associated with lower risk of diabetes. (A meta-analysis is a statistical technique for combining and analysing the findings of independent trials.)

A recent study by Dr Shilpa Bhupathiraju, a nutrition expert at Harvard University in the USA, looked at three large groups with similar characteristics and found that those who increased their coffee drinking by around one and a half cups of coffee per day had an 11 per cent lower risk of developing Type 2 diabetes over the following four years.[12]

Metformin may be prescribed

In some people who are pre-diabetic, but whose efforts to keep the HbA1c down have not been successful, the biguanide drug metformin may be prescribed. We will consider this drug in Chapter 9 (*Drugs for Type 2 diabetes*).

Management of your diabetes

Once Type 2 diabetes is diagnosed by your GP, the ongoing management will usually be carried out at the practice, either by the GP and by the practice nurse or by a designated diabetes nurse.

Receiving the diagnosis is a life-changing event. It certainly should be, because the first thing that ought to take place is that you are given help to understand the nature of Type 2 diabetes and all of its implications. It varies from practice to practice as to how this is done. In some the GP will do this over several appointments. In others the practice nurse or diabetic nurse will sit down and go through everything, supplying educational leaflets and literature and guiding you to sites on the Internet.

In other practices there may be specially arranged educational courses within the practice, at the hospital or in a health centre, and meetings with other patients. These are part of the DESMOND (Diabetes Education and Self Management for Ongoing and Newly Diagnosed) programme. This specialises in helping people with Type 2 diabetes to self-manage their condition effectively. We will look at this further in Chapter 8 (*Lifestyle changes to treat Type 2 diabetes*). The psychological aspect of coming to terms with the diagnosis and how the condition will affect your life is something that ought to be covered in any educational programme about diabetes. We shall also be looking at this in more detail with some strategies, in Chapter 10 (*Using the Life Cycle with Type 2 diabetes*).

Your GP or diabetes nurse may want to keep a close check on you to begin with, perhaps weekly or fortnightly, to monitor blood pressure, weight and perhaps feet and how well the blood-glucose is doing.

Glucose monitoring

This is the fundamental measurement of how well you are managing your diabetes. This is something that the patient does regularly him or herself. Your GP will inform you about how to do this and will advise on the exact procedures.

With Type 2 diabetes there are basically two methods of glucose monitoring:

- urine testing
- blood testing for glucose and ketones.

Your GP will explain how your treatment may be altered according to test levels. You will be fully involved in this and not just the recipient of drugs.

Urine testing

For the majority of Type 2 diabetics who are being treated with diet or diet and oral hypoglycaemic drugs (except gliflozins, the SGLT2 inhibitors – see Chapter 9: *Drugs for Type 2 diabetes* – that always cause glucose to appear in the urine) urine tests are adequate for monitoring the condition.

This test depends on the fact that there is a renal threshold at which glucose spills into the urine. This is generally at a blood-glucose level of 10.0 mmol/l, so if the blood-glucose is consistently below this no glucose will appear. If you get consistently negative tests it indicates that your blood-glucose is not getting up to 10.0 mmol/l, which means that a lot of the readings will be below that. This is regarded as being reasonable control. If you get positive readings, then your GP will want to check blood-glucose or HbA1c levels and possibly adjust treatment.

Test strips are used, which are prescribed by your GP. The test strips have a number of boxes with different colours. The test strip will change to a colour that can then be compared against the code on the side of the test strip container, to give a reading the equivalent of the blood-glucose at that time.

To do the test the strip can be dipped into the stream of urine or dipped into a specimen that has been freshly passed. You can test at various times of the day to see how the urine test relates to meals. The morning test should always be done using a fresh sample, which means avoiding the first passage of urine and waiting half an hour before doing the first test. This ensures that you are not measuring an accumulated sample from overnight.

KETONES

Ketones are acid chemicals produced in the body if the body has insufficient insulin effect so it cannot move glucose into the cells. As a result the body will start to burn fat and the process of gluconeogenesis will be put into operation. This converts fatty acids into glucose (see Chapter 3: *Metabolism and what goes wrong in diabetes*).

A high level of ketones is one of the complications of Type 1 diabetes (which we shall look at in Chapter 7: *The complications of diabetes*), which can lead to ketoacidosis. It can also occur in advanced Type 2 diabetes.

Finding ketones in the urine is always a sign that the diabetes treatment needs altering. If you find this, contact your GP.

Testing strips similar to the urine glucose test strips are used and they can be prescribed by your GP.

Blood testing for glucose and ketones

This test is most often done by pricking a finger with a needle to produce a drop of blood. The blood is pressed onto a test strip, which is then inserted into a glucose meter that also measures ketones. The test strips are prescribed by the GP, but the glucose meter may have to be purchased. Some diabetic centres may have them available, but it varies.

There are two methods used, but you may need advice about which glucose meter to use. Your GP or diabetic nurse may be able to help. Alternatively, you could check the Diabetes UK website, which has useful information about them.

There are two types of meters:

- colour-testing-strip meters – these have a small area on the test strip that changes colour when the blood is added. This is inserted into the meter, which gives a reading from the colour change.
- chemical-retain-strip meters – the test strip does not change colour, but a chemical reaction takes place that gives a reading when inserted into the meter. This is more accurate and most meters tend to use this method nowadays.

Blood-glucose monitoring is most useful if a person has diabetes that is harder to control. The glucose readings may be used to adjust the dose of insulin, if this is being used. Your GP and diabetic nurse will give full instructions on this.

Treatment of Type 2 diabetes

The whole aim of treatment is to keep the blood-glucose under control, meaning keeping it in the range that you would expect in people who do not have diabetes.

The treatment options are twofold.

1. Lifestyle changes:

- diet
- weight control
- exercise.

2. Medication: using the drug metformin and other hypoglycaemic drugs as needed, or insulin if this is ultimately indicated.

We will be considering all of these treatment options in Chapter 8 (*Lifestyle changes to treat Type 2 diabetes*) and Chapter 9 (*Drugs to treat Type 2 diabetes*).

A tailored diabetic plan

Do not worry; the management of diabetes is not just up to you, the patient. There are certain things that should be looked at on a regular basis, and which you can expect to be available. The National Institute for Health and Clinical Excellence (NICE) has suggested that there should be a tailored diabetic plan for every person with diabetes, which includes several things that ought to be looked at on an annual basis.

Your GP is currently remunerated for doing these and has to record them in order to achieve payment for the Quality Outcome Framework (or QOF) points.

Diabetes UK has drawn up a list of factors that should be covered at an annual examination. These include:

1. Blood-glucose monitoring by HbA1c test

This gives a good assessment of what the blood-glucose has been doing over the preceding two or three months.

The aim of good control of the diabetes is to get the HbA1c level down to 48.0 mmol/mol (6.5 per cent). This would be considered good control, although some people may prefer their numbers to be closer to that of non-diabetics, which would be 41.0 mmol/l (5.9 per cent) or less. As I outlined earlier, HbA1c levels between 6.0 per cent and 6.4 per cent would indicate that the person has pre-diabetes and is at increased risk of developing diabetes.

The two large-scale studies that I will detail in Chapter 7 (*The complications of diabetes*) – the UK Prospective Diabetes Study (UKPDS) and the Diabetes Control and Complications Trial (DCCT), both demonstrated that improving HbA1c by 1 per cent (or 11.0 mmol/mol) for people with Type 1 diabetes *or* Type 2 diabetes cuts the risk of micro-vascular complications by 25 per cent. This means that the risk of retinopathy, neuropathy and nephropathy would all be reduced.

Other research[13] on people with Type 2 diabetes showed that reducing the HbA1c by 1 per cent brought about a reduction in risk of:

- cataract by 19 per cent
- heart failure by 16 per cent
- amputation rate by 43 per cent.

2. Lipids

Most people know that a high cholesterol level in the blood is not good for you. It can increase the risk of heart disease or of having a stroke. It is not just the level of cholesterol that matters, however, but the relative balance between good cholesterol and bad cholesterol. Essentially the lower the level of bad cholesterol, the lower your risk.

Cholesterol is a type of waxy, fat substance that is found in all of the body's cells. It is, in fact, an important substance for the body, but you just do not want too much of it. Cholesterol is carried around the bloodstream in packets called lipoproteins. The 'lipo' is the inside part of the package and consists of fat, the 'protein' is the outer part. There are two types of lipoprotein that carry your cholesterol – low-density lipoprotein (or LDL), commonly known as bad cholesterol, and high-density lipoprotein (or HDL), commonly thought of as good cholesterol.

The blood test for fats in the blood is called a lipid profile. It measures HDL cholesterol, LDL cholesterol, total cholesterol and triglycerides, which are another type of blood fat. If the triglyceride level is raised it is another risk factor. These levels are measured in millimoles per litre, mmol/l.

It is desirable for the total cholesterol to be under 5.0 mmol/l and for the cholesterol to HDL ratio to be less than five.

3. Blood pressure

Hypertension puts the person at risk of several problems, so its control is of paramount importance. It tends not to cause any symptoms, so you will not know that you have a problem with it until you have your blood pressure taken.

Your GP or the practice nurse will measure your blood pressure using a calibrated and regularly maintained machine. Practices have all of their sphygmomanometers calibrated, so that all practitioners and nurses are measuring blood pressures with the same accuracy.

The blood pressure is usually taken seated. A blood pressure cuff is wrapped around the upper arm and it is then inflated. It will either be done with an automated machine or by using an aneroid sphygmomanometer and a stethoscope.

4. Eye examination

Eyesight should be checked at the annual examination. There should also be a retinopathy screening. This may be done at the ophthalmology department at the hospital or arranged with a local optician. Drops are usually needed to dilate the pupil. It requires a photograph to be taken of each retina. This will act as a record for future comparison, to assess the development of retinopathy or worsening of it.

5. Foot examination

This involves looking at the skin colour, the state and integrity of the skin and the nerve supply of the skin. The doctor will check for touch and temperature sensation. These are important because of the risks of injury or burning if you cannot feel when you are being touched or when extreme heat or cold is applied to the feet. An example of an injury would be stubbing a toe, and a burn could occur from a burst hot water bottle.

The examination also involves checking the toes, the blood supply and the nails and areas around the nails for evidence of infection or alteration in the shape of the feet, which may occur if the joints become damaged.

6. Kidney function

This will involve urine testing for albumin and blood testing for creatinine. See the section on kidney complications in Chapter 7 (*The complications of diabetes*).

7. Weight check

This should be done to check on:

- height and weight, to calculate the body mass index (BMI). See Chapter 8 (*Lifestyle changes to treat Type 2 diabetes*).
- waist–hips ratio with the aim to reduce waist measurement to less than 80 centimetres for women or 94 centimetres for men.

8. Check on smoking habit

If advice on stopping is needed, then it will be given. See Chapter 8 (*Lifestyle changes to treat Type 2 diabetes*).

9. A review of your management plan

Everyone should have a plan made when he or she is diagnosed or when visiting the general practice for the first time to have his or her diabetes monitored. This will be a review of how well everything is being done and how well the control of weight, blood pressure and HbA1c has been. If there have been complications, then medication may need altering and referral to specialists may be made.

10. Specialist referral for pregnant women with diabetes

If you have become pregnant, then referral to a specialist in diabetic care as well as to an obstetric unit should be made. The care of a woman with diabetes is crucial to her well-being and the well-being of her baby.

11. Review of psychological well-being

There will be questions about sleep, mood and general emotions to determine how well the person is doing and whether there is any problem with anxiety, insomnia or depression. Appropriate counselling or medication may be required.

It is a good idea to sit and think ahead of the annual visit about any concerns that you have. This could relate to general health, risk of other conditions or difficulties that you may be having in other areas of your life, such as your sex life. Do not be at all embarrassed; you can ask your doctor anything.

DRIVING AND TYPE 2 DIABETES

- Type 2 diabetes will not cause you to lose your licence.
- You only have to notify DVLA if you are on insulin, sulphonylureas or glinides.
- You should notify DVLA if you have eye or nerve complications.
- If you have notified them about such complications or about being on insulin, sulphonylureas or glinides, DVLA will seek medical information and issue a three-year licence, provided your blood-glucose measurements do not show any hypoglycaemic episodes (for this you will need twice-a-day readings recorded over three months).
- The three-year licence will require a questionnaire from you and possibly a medical examination by your GP before renewal.
- If you have a group 2 licence (for lorries and buses) you will have to be free of hypoglycaemic attacks for 12 months preceding the application.
- You would be advised to notify your medical insurance upon being diagnosed with diabetes.
- See DVLA in the Directory of useful addresses.

Chapter 7

The complications of diabetes

The complications of diabetes make early diagnosis so important. The longer it remains undiagnosed, the longer the elevated blood-glucose will have been causing damage to the body's various systems. It is important to keep diabetes under control to limit further damage and complications.

The good news is that you can live life very well and you can avoid complications by managing your diabetes efficiently. There have been two very large studies, one from the UK and one from the USA, which looked at reducing the risk of complications.

The Diabetes Control and Complications Trial (DCCT) was a major clinical study conducted from 1983 to 1993 in the USA that looked at patients with Type 1 diabetes. It showed that good control limits the risk of complications.

Of more interest to us in terms of Type 2 diabetes was the UK Prospective Diabetes Study (UKPDS) which was a randomised, multi-centre trial of blood-glucose reducing treatments in 5,102 patients with newly diagnosed Type 2 diabetes. It ran for 20 years, between 1977 and 1997, and showed conclusively that the complications of

Type 2 diabetes could be reduced by improving blood-glucose and by maintaining good blood pressure control.

Figure 14: **The places of the body where diabetic complications can occur**

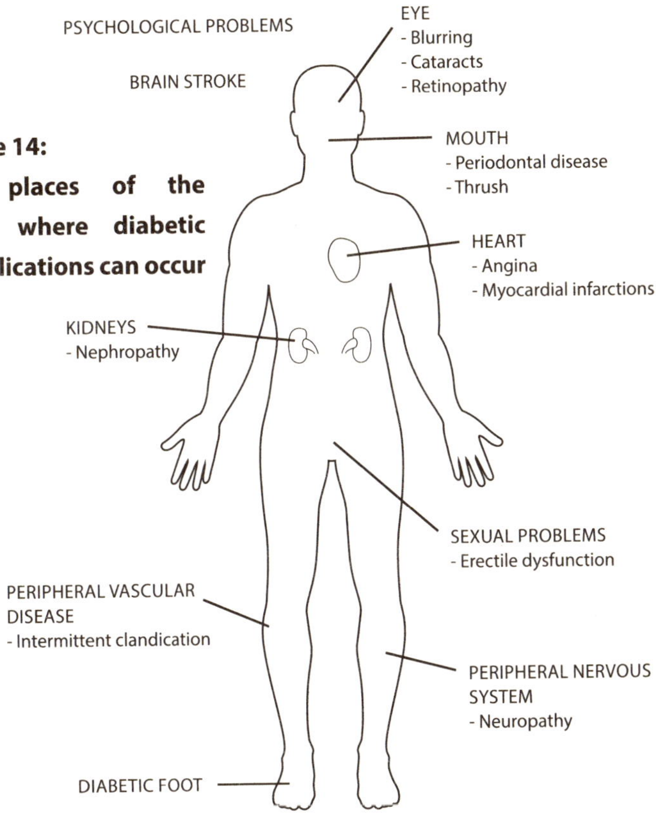

General treatment of all complications

This will involve treating the symptoms of the complications, but most importantly, the aim is to gain as good control of the diabetes as possible. That means keeping blood-glucose and blood pressure under control, ideally by:

- keeping weight under control and maintaining a BMI within the normal range. The BMI is essentially giving an estimation of human body fat, although it does not actually measure fat.
- eating a healthy diet.
- taking regular exercise.
- avoiding or stopping smoking.
- keeping alcohol intake within safe limits.
- having regular reviews of your diabetes.

Metabolic complications

Predominantly, this is about blood-glucose. The level can cause problems if it rises too high as a result of the condition not being managed adequately or due to an acute illness, like an infection that will often cause the blood-glucose to go out of control. Conversely, the level can drop too low as a result of treatment.

Hypoglycaemia

'Hypo' means low, so hypoglycaemia means low blood-sugar. This happens if the blood-sugar drops below 4.0 mmol/l. This level means that the body does not have enough glucose to provide the energy needed for activity.

This can cause any of the following symptoms:

- feeling faint

- shakiness
- sweating
- blurred vision
- hunger
- difficulty concentrating
- headache
- mood change
- increasing drowsiness
- unconsciousness.

Hypoglycaemia is more likely in Type 1 diabetes as a result of too much insulin, but it can occur with too much oral medication in Type 2 diabetes, or if there has been excessive exertion, insufficient food intake or too much alcohol. And of course, it can occur in Type 2 diabetes if insulin is being taken as part of the medication regime.

Hyperglycaemia

'Hyper' means high, so hyperglycaemia means high blood-glucose. This is defined as above 7.0 mmol/l before a meal or above 8.5 mmol/l two hours after a meal. It can happen if too much carbohydrate has been taken in, if there is an underlying infection or if medication has been missed.

This can cause the following symptoms:

- excess urination
- excess thirst

- headache
- lethargy
- drowsiness.

Ketoacidosis

In Type 1 diabetes the blood-glucose can go so high that it causes a dangerous complication called diabetic ketoacidosis, DKA. This is a state in which the blood-glucose rises very high, above 20.0 mmol/l and the blood becomes acidic and accumulates ketones, which are the breakdown products of fat. This is because the body automatically uses gluconeogenesis to build glucose from fatty acids, as explained in Chapter 3 (*Metabolism and what goes wrong in diabetes*). Ketoacidosis requires emergency treatment.

It can cause the following symptoms:

- extreme weakness
- possibly unconsciousness and coma
- rapid breathing, called air hunger or Kussmaul breathing. This is because the body tries to blow off carbon dioxide in order to lower the acidity of the blood.
- nausea and vomiting
- acetone breath
- dehydration
- low potassium level in the blood, which can cause muscle cramps, weakness, nausea or vomiting, and palpitations.

Ketoacidosis is rare in Type 2 diabetes because the body is still producing some insulin, albeit the body does not react adequately to it. It can occur if there is a severe infection or trauma or if the body is under extreme physical exertion. It can also occur in poorly controlled, long-standing Type 2 diabetes. It is a serious condition with a mortality rate of ten per cent.

Hyperosmolar hyperglycaemic state

This is another state that can arise from excess blood-glucose. This is also a medical emergency that needs hospital treatment. It can occur very rapidly, within hours.

'Hyper' means high and 'osmolar' refers to the concentration in the blood. In other words, the blood gets extremely concentrated with blood-glucose. The levels can be much higher than ketoacidosis, 33.0 mmol/l or more. It is not associated with the same acidity as ketoacidosis, but there is still breakdown of fats to produce ketones.

It can cause the following symptoms:

- excess urination
- excess thirst
- drowsiness and even coma
- cramps
- dehydration.

The rapid breathing or air hunger of Kussmaul breathing does not occur.

This condition often takes days to build up. It is commonest in Type 2 diabetics whose control has been neglected. It can occur in diabetics living alone who have not cared for themselves or who have fallen ill and stopped being able to care for themselves. It can occur in residential homes if staff are unaware of the diabetes or of the nature of and potential problems associated with this complication.

Lactic acidosis

This is a state in which the blood becomes excessively acidic, with a pH of 7.25 or less (normal pH is 7.4) and is caused by a build up of lactic acid. This is usually cleared from the system by the kidneys, liver and muscles. In Type 2 diabetes it is a rare side effect of the drug metformin, occurring in one in 30,000 patients.

It can produce the following symptoms:

- tiredness
- weakness
- muscle pains
- shortness of breath
- stomach pains
- feeling cold
- dizziness
- developing a slow or irregular heartbeat.

It can be extremely dangerous and if these symptoms come on suddenly and severely and you are taking metformin, treat it as an emergency and call medical aid. It needs blood tests to diagnose it and treatment in a hospital.

Cardiovascular complications

Raised blood-glucose over several years damages arterial blood vessels and worsens arteriosclerosis, or hardening of the arteries.

It is not all about blood-glucose, though

It is important to appreciate that it is not just the blood-glucose that matters. The evidence from research is that raised cholesterol and high blood pressure are also significant factors in producing arteriosclerosis. Indeed, reducing blood pressure and lowering cholesterol can prevent three times as many heart attacks and strokes than reducing blood-glucose alone.[14]

It is well established that diabetes is an independent risk factor for stroke and heart disease. This means that even when one allows for the fact that obesity, raised cholesterol and hypertension are more common in diabetes, even when these factors are all controlled, the risk is still twice that of a non-diabetic person. This makes it all the more important for diabetics to do all that they can to keep their sugar levels under control.

KEY POINTS

- Diabetes increases the risk of having a heart attack by two to five times.
- Diabetes increases the risk of having a stroke by two to three times.
- Reducing blood pressure and cholesterol prevents three times as many heart attacks and strokes as lowering blood-glucose alone.

We are now in a position to consider the complications of the cardiovascular system. These arise from arteriosclerosis – the hardening of the large arteries that supply the various parts of the body.

Heart

The coronary arteries supply the heart muscle (the myocardium). Partial blockage will cause angina pectoris. This is the state in which ischaemia occurs, leading to cramp pains in the chest and often down the left arm, which occurs on exertion and is relieved by resting.

A myocardial infarction is the death of part of the heart muscle caused by complete blockage of a coronary artery. This is the correct name for a heart attack. It always needs treatment as it can cause heart failure or even sudden death.

Warning signs of a heart attack

If you develop sudden severe chest pain that makes you feel clammy and nauseated then you may be having a heart attack. If you have a history of angina and have a supply of glyceryl trinitrate (GTN) tablets or a nitrolingual spray (the usual treatments for angina) then try one tablet or one or two sprays, then repeat after five minutes. If there is no improvement, call for medical aid.

If you have never had angina and experience such a pain, call for medical aid.

Brain

Arteriosclerosis affecting the cerebral arteries supplying the brain can cause a stroke. This is the name given for a 'brain attack'.

A reversible stroke that completely resolves in 24 hours or less is called a mini-stroke or a transient cerebral ischaemic attack, or TCIA.

A major stroke persists for longer and may never recover completely. It is caused by either ischaemia or a haemorrhage in one side of the brain, resulting in partial or complete paralysis of the other side of the body.

A subarachnoid haemorrhage is a third, less common type of stroke, which tends to have a totally different presentation from other types of stroke. It is the result of a bleed from an aneurysm, a little 'balloon' that forms on some brain vessels. The bleed in this case is between the arachnoid membrane and the pia membrane. These are two of the meninges, or the membranes, which cover the brain. (These membranes can become inflamed in meningitis, which is of viral or bacterial origin.)

A stroke is a major life event and if the person suffers from one and survives it, there may be considerable disability for years or even for the remainder of life. It is also a significant cause of death. The important thing to appreciate is that strokes are all preventable, which means that good diabetic control is of paramount importance.

KEY POINTS

- Eighty per cent of strokes are ischaemic.
- Fifteen per cent of strokes are haemorrhagic.
- Five per cent of strokes are subarachnoid.

Warning symptoms of a stroke and the FAST test

There is no typical stroke. There are many variants, depending upon which part of the brain has been affected. The most important thing to appreciate is that a stroke is a medical emergency. It is vital to get help for yourself, if you think you are having a stroke, or for someone who seems to be having a stroke. Speed is essential.

The Stroke Association has a campaign that you may have seen on television, on posters or in magazines and newspapers. It is a simple mnemonic that alerts you to the things to look for and the action you must take.

FAST stands for:

- FACIAL weakness – ask the person to smile. Look to see if the mouth is drooping on one side.
- ARM weakness – can the person raise both arms?
- SPEECH problems – can the person speak clearly, without slurring? Do they understand what you are saying?
- TIME TO CALL the emergency number 999!

Quite simply, if the person fails any of these tests there is enough evidence to suspect he or she is having a stroke. The faster you get help, the better the prospect of minimising damage to the brain. This will improve his or her chances of recovery. It may even save his or her life.

Peripheral vascular disease

The large peripheral arteries supplying the limbs can be affected by arteriosclerosis to produce intermittent claudication, which is painful cramp in the legs on walking. This can occur after only a few hundred yards, when the person must stop in order to let the cramp disappear. The smaller blood vessels may also be affected, putting the individual at risk of developing gangrene, as we shall consider in the section on the foot.

Treatment of cardiovascular complications

Prevention of complications is a fundamental aim in diabetic control, as is prevention of further deterioration of a complication if it has already started to develop.

Treating raised cholesterol with statins and raised blood pressure with one or more anti-hypertensive drugs is of prime importance.

If established artery blockages have occurred, then it may be possible to widen them with balloon angioplasty, in which a thin catheter is inserted into an artery and threaded along the vessel to the area of blockage where a tiny balloon is inflated to widen the blocked segment. Alternatively, a catheter may be used to insert a stent, a miniature wire-framed cylinder into the blockage to open it up and keep it permanently open.

If the blockage is extensive, then further surgery to replace the diseased segments with healthy veins from another part of the body may be needed. In the case of the heart this is called a coronary artery bypass graft, CABG. This procedure can replace, one, two or even three arteries to the heart. Similar surgery may be available for peripheral vascular disease affecting the arteries in the legs to produce major intermittent claudication.

Kidney complications

As we saw in Chapter 4 (*The symptoms of diabetes and how they come about*), the kidneys are highly important organs needed to filter the blood and remove toxins, among other important functions. If we reconsider the functions of the kidneys, then we can see what the results of kidney damage will be.

Normal functions of the kidneys

- Filter the blood and remove waste products, such as urea and creatinine, and the clearance of some drugs from the body.
- Prevent build up of fluid in the body.
- Maintain levels of electrolytes, such as sodium, potassium and phosphate.
- Produce hormones that:
    - regulate blood pressure.
    - make red blood cells.
    - keep bones strong by maintaining calcium levels.

Kidney damage will result in:

- diminished filtering and removal of waste products so that the body is poisoned by these waste products.
- fluid may accumulate in the body, causing swollen ankles and feet.
- the electrolyte balance of sodium, potassium, chloride and phosphorus may be impaired. This can affect other organs like the heart.
- kidney disease, which raises blood pressure to cause hypertension.
- anaemia due to failure to produce enough red blood cells.

Kidney damage can cause:

- osteoporosis causing bone loss and increased susceptibility to fractured bones.

Diabetic nephropathy

This is the name given to kidney disease as a result of diabetes. It can occur in both diabetes Type 1 and Type 2. This will affect 40 per cent of people with diabetes.

Damage to the glomeruli – the microscopic knots of blood vessels that form part of the nephron, the filtering unit of the kidney – occurs because of high blood pressure, hardening of the arterioles and the raised blood-glucose (causing AGEs, as outlined earlier). The glomeruli get blocked and no longer work. As a result, the tubules attached to each blocked glomerulus stop working. The overall filtering ability of the kidney gets progressively reduced.

This is rather like a tea strainer having extra holes punched in it, so that it filters less effectively allowing larger particles to pass through into the teacup. In the case of the kidney, the larger holes allow substances that are normally retained in the blood to get passed into the urine. The first thing of importance is protein, which leaks into the urine.

When the doctor or nurse tests the urine they not only test for glucose but test to detect the presence of albumen, a particular type of protein. If it is present in the urine it is called microalbuminuria. This may be a sign of kidney disease, though it may also be present if there is a urinary tract infection. A urine culture would then be needed to exclude this.

If no infection is present, then regular urine testing is needed to monitor the urine to assess ongoing progression of kidney disease. Urine testing would indicate greater quantities of protein to be present. This would indicate further loss of glomeruli and nephron filtering units, so even more protein would leak into the urine. This can be visible as frothy urine.

KEY POINTS

- All people with diabetes should be screened for kidney disease once a year.
- The symptoms of diabetic nephropathy may only occur in the later stages of the condition.
- It is a minority of people with diabetes Type 2 who will require renal transplantation or need dialysis.

Symptoms of diabetic nephropathy

In the early stages there are no symptoms. As the diabetic nephropathy worsens and symptoms become apparent, together with blood and urine tests confirming the diagnosis, it is called chronic kidney disease (CKD).

The following symptoms may start to occur:

- nausea or vomiting.
- tiredness as a result of a lack of oxygen in the blood.
- fluid retention with swelling of the ankles, feet, lower legs or hands.

- darker urine, caused by blood in the urine.
- becoming short of breath, when climbing the stairs, for instance.
- muscle cramps.
- itching skin.
- increasing blood pressure.

Stages of diabetic nephropathy

Diabetic patients should all have regular assessments of their kidney function, at least once a year.

One of the main tests is the estimated Glomerular Filtration Rate, or eGFR. This is a blood test that assesses how much blood is filtered and cleared of waste products per minute. The reading is given in millilitres per minute (ml/min). The eGFR is worked out by measuring the level of creatinine in the blood. This is a breakdown product of muscle that is excreted in the urine. As kidney function deteriorates the blood level of creatinine rises.

The eGFR in normal health is 90 or more ml/min. With worsening diabetic nephropathy, meaning worsening kidney function that level drops.

Five stages of diabetic nephropathy are recognised. It may take 20 years for someone's kidney function to deteriorate from stage 1 to stage 5.

Stage 1: normal – eGFR of greater than 90 ml/min with other evidence of chronic kidney damage, such as albumin or blood in the urine, or an abnormality of the kidney shown on ultrasound or X-ray examination.

Stage 2: mild impairment – eGFR of 60–89 ml/min with other evidence of chronic kidney damage.
Stage 3a: moderate impairment – eGFR of 45–59 ml/min.
Stage 3b: moderate impairment – eGFR of 30–44 ml/min.
Stage 4: severe impairment – eGFR of 15–29 ml/min.
Stage 5: established renal failure (ERF), also known as end stage renal disease (ESRD) – eGFR of less than 15 ml/min or on dialysis.

Figure 15 shows how the five stages relate to diminishing kidney function and the progressive development of symptoms.

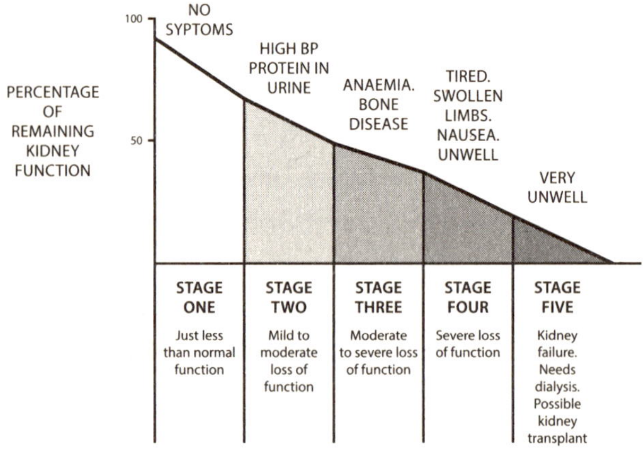

Figure 15: The five stages of diabetic nephropathy/chronic kidney disease

People with stages 3, 4 and 5, defined as an eGFR of less than 60 ml/min are said to have chronic kidney disease, or CKD. People often feel quite well even with an eGFR of only 30 ml/min. Below that eGFR, symptoms are certainly expected.

Treatment of diabetic nephropathy

The aim, as with all complications is to minimise further damage by maintaining as good control of the diabetes as possible.

If there is hypertension (raised blood pressure), then this should be controlled as well as possible. In particular, anti-hypertensive drugs belonging to the angiotensin-converting enzyme (ACE) inhibiter group of drugs or to the angiotensin receptor blocker (ARB) group of drugs may help, because they have been shown to reduce blood pressure and also preserve kidney function.

If the kidneys have become so damaged that kidney failure and established renal failure is present, with macroalbuminuria (large amounts of protein in the urine), then kidney transplantation may be considered. This may be dependent upon whether there is an available donor of a single kidney.

A live donated kidney has a better chance of success than one donated from someone who has died. The best match possible will be from a family member. Rejection of a donated organ is always a potential problem and the person receiving the kidney will have to be on immune-suppressive drugs to prevent this rejection for the rest of their life.

The actual operation takes about four hours. The kidney may not be properly functional for several weeks so renal dialysis will be needed until then. Renal dialysis is a process in which the filtering function of the kidneys is done artificially. There are two methods:

1. Haemodialysis

A haemodialysis machine is essentially an artificial kidney. Blood is removed via a cannula and tubing and circulated through a machine that filters, cleans and returns the blood to the body. This takes about four hours to do and is required about three times a week. It usually needs to be done in a renal unit in hospital.

2. Peritoneal dialysis

This is a more convenient method, which even allows people to have it done at home. Clean dialysis fluid is dribbled through a tube into the abdomen. Waste from the blood enters the abdominal cavity and the dialysis fluid. The fluid can be exchanged several times a day or during the night using a small dialysis machine.

Eye complications

These complications come about because the eyes, like the kidneys, have an extremely rich blood supply of tiny arterioles and capillaries. There are various eye problems that can complicate Type 2 diabetes.

Figure 16 shows the various parts of the eye. Essentially, the eye is a spherical camera. The muscular sclera, the white of the eye, forms the sphere and is continuous with the transparent front of the eye, the cornea. Light rays enter the eye and are focused by the lens onto the retina, which is the light-sensitive 'seeing' membrane at the back of the eye. The amount of light let into the eye is determined by the reflex actions that govern the movement of the iris and the shape of the lens; the focus is adjusted by the ciliary muscles.

There are two fluids in the eye, the aqueous humour at the front of the eye between the lens and the cornea, and the jelly-like vitreous humour behind the lens.

The retina has two types of cells called rods and cones. There are about 120 million rods in the eye and about six to seven million cones, which are colour sensitive. The rods are distributed about the whole retina, but the cones are predominantly situated around the centre of the eye, the part called the macula.

Signals from the eye are transmitted to the brain via the optic nerve, which is the second of the twelve cranial nerves.

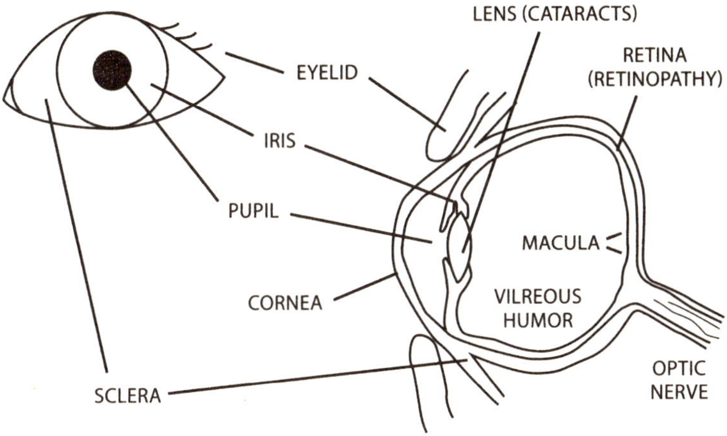

Figure 16: The human eye and the areas that are at risk of the complications of diabetes

Blurring of vision

This often occurs when the condition is diagnosed and treatment is started. The problem starts because the raised blood-glucose results in water coming out of the lens at the front of the eye, so that it becomes dehydrated. When treatment is started with tablets (blurring does not tend to occur just with diet control, since the rectification is gentler) the blood-glucose will drop relatively quickly. Water then gets resorbed into the lens to hydrate it. This of course changes its shape and alters the focal length, so that the image becomes blurred.

This is usually completely reversible and just requires a time to adjust. This may take several weeks and it is best to be patient. If you rush to the optician to change a prescription for spectacles you may find that the situation changes again soon after.

Cataracts

These are cloudy opacities that form in the lens of the eye. The cloudiness that forms in the lens is rather like looking through frosted glass. They can occur in normal health and become commoner with increasing age, but are definitely more common in people with both Type 1 and Type 2 diabetes. Overall, people with diabetes are 60 per cent more likely to develop cataracts.

Smoking is an additional risk factor, so it is important that people with Type 2 diabetes should not smoke if they want to avoid this complication.

A cataract may form in one or both eyes, but not necessarily at the same rate. Most cataracts worsen, especially in middle age, if you have Type 2 diabetes.

People may notice difficulty with reading, but also driving at night when car headlights shine straight in the eyes and the light rays get scattered by the cataracts to cause dazzling.

There is, as yet, nothing that will reverse a cataract. For diabetics with them, keeping good control of the condition may prevent rapid deterioration. If it does not, there is a simple operation, which can be performed under local anaesthesia, to remove the lens containing the cataract and replace it with an artificial lens. The operation usually takes 20–30 minutes. It is a keyhole operation in which a small tube is inserted into the eye to suck the cataract out. A plastic lens implant is then put in its place. The plastic lens implant is placed in the capsule of the lens.

Cataract surgery is regarded as one of the safest and most effective of operations, with the risk of a serious problem being only one per cent.

Glaucoma

This is a condition that can occur in anyone, but it is more common in diabetics, especially if there is diabetic retinopathy (see below).

In glaucoma there is an increase in pressure within the eye because of an increase in fluid within the eye. This increase in pressure can damage the delicate retina and the optic nerve – the seeing part of the eye – at the back of the eyeball.

The eye actually produces fluid that circulates around the lens. This is then drained into the bloodstream. If there is blockage to the flow of fluid by, for example, new blood vessels, as happens in diabetic retinopathy, then the fluid accumulates in the eye increasing the pressure.

There may be no symptoms, which is one of the reasons that all diabetic people should have regular eye checks. Some people do have deteriorating vision, so this should never be ignored. It is always sensible to check it out at the first sign of a change in vision.

Some people with glaucoma experience a sort of tunnel vision in that they seem to lose the outer parts of their visual fields. Classically, glaucoma causes haloes to appear around lights. This should always be followed by investigation and probably assessment by an optician or ophthalmologist, an eye specialist.

The treatment usually consists of eye drops and sometimes a special type of diuretic (water removing pill) to reduce the pressure. In some people there is an operation called a partial iridectomy, which involves removing a small wedge of the iris of the eye, the coloured part around the pupil. This permits the circulation of fluid within the eye and drops the pressure.

Diabetic retinopathy

The retina is richly supplied with blood vessels. These, like the blood vessels that form the glomeruli in the kidneys, can be damaged by excess blood-glucose, hardening of the blood vessels and high blood pressure. Their walls can become weakened and bulge out. When examined closely by an optician or by a doctor using an instrument called an ophthalmoscope to look inside the eye, tiny balloon bulges called microaneurysms may be seen on the blood vessels on the retina. Some of these can burst to cause tiny haemorrhages. They can also leak to accumulate fluid on the retina. These can then harden, like small scars, on the retinal surface. These are called hard exudates.

Changes on the retina of the eye are called retinopathy. These are regularly checked by your doctor and have to be followed up to assess deterioration. Good diabetes control must be aimed to prevent deterioration.

Retinopathy is uncommon in the first five years of diabetes. It becomes more common the longer you have it, so that after 25 years about 90 per cent of people with Type 2 diabetes will have some degree of retinopathy.

Symptoms of retinopathy

There may be no symptoms in the early stages of retinopathy. The following may all occur:

- sudden blurring
- sudden deterioration of vision

- floaters and spots before the eyes
- pain in one or both eyeballs.

Stages of retinopathy

There are four ever more extensive stages of retinopathy.

1. Background retinopathy

This is mild and does not affect vision. There may be some tiny leaks of fluid and tiny microaneurysms and tiny haemorrhages on various parts of the retina. These will be seen as tiny dots and blots on the retina on eye examination with an ophthalmoscope.

2. Pre-proliferative retinopathy

This is more extensive than background retinopathy. There may be some exudates, which look like tiny blobs of fat on the retina. There are signs of blood flow becoming restricted, but no evidence that new blood vessels are growing.

3. Maculopathy

This is when there is damage to your macula. This is serious because it affects the very central part of vision, so the person may not see straight ahead and may not be able to read because he or she can only see with the peripheral parts of his or her visual fields.

4. Proliferative retinopathy

This occurs when damaged blood vessels are stimulated by chemicals called growth factors. These stimulate new blood vessel growth from the damaged blood vessels. Thus the blood vessels are proliferating, hence the name of proliferative retinopathy. This is the eye's attempt to repair the damage. Unfortunately, these new blood vessels are delicate and friable, meaning that they burst and bleed easily. This can seriously impair vision.

Proliferative retinopathy can result in:

- Retinal detachment – when the retina is pulled off the back of the eye. This can occur because of increased fibre deposition that takes place in retinopathy.
- Retinal detachment is considered a medical emergency and needs urgent treatment. It can cause sudden partial visual loss. It can also lead to total blindness in the eye. It is more common in:
    - those aged 50–75 years.
    - short-sighted people.
- Vitreous haemorrhage – when there is bleeding into the vitreous humour. This may cause sudden disturbance or loss of vision or floaters.
- Glaucoma (see page 125) – if new vessels interfere with the circulation of fluid, fluid will accumulate and increase pressure within the eyeball.

Treatment of retinopathy

Recent research suggests that statins used to reduce cholesterol levels may also be helpful in reducing nerve damage and retinopathy in diabetics.[15]

The mainstay of therapy these days is laser treatment. It can seal off bleeding vessels or vessels that look as if they are about to burst. It can also prevent new vessel growth, hence reduce the proliferative changes that take place. It cannot restore vision that has been lost, but it may prevent further deterioration.

Macular oedema may be helped by laser treatment, but it can be very difficult to treat. Injections directly into the area of the macula may be needed.

If the vitreous becomes hard and rubbery, losing its usual jelly-like consistency, it can shrink. This produces a vitreous detachment, where it pulls away from the retina. The danger then is that the retina is not being kept in place and may lift off as a retinal detachment. A vitrectomy operation to remove the vitreous may then be done in a specialist unit. This involves removing the vitreous and replacing it with an oil-based fluid.

The NHS report that:

- 1,280 new cases of blindness are caused by diabetic retinopathy are reported each year in England.
- an additional 4,200 people in England are thought to be at risk of retinopathy-related vision loss.

Nerve complications

The nervous system is the body's main communication system. It is customary to consider it as having the following three parts:

1. The central nervous system, consisting of the brain, the cranial nerves (nerves of the head and neck that come directly out from the brain, rather than from the spine) and the spinal cord.

2. The peripheral nervous system, consisting of the nerves to the various parts of the body.
3. The autonomic nervous system, consisting of two components:
   - Sympathetic nervous system that prepares you for fight or flight.
   - Parasympathetic nervous system that controls the involuntary functions of our bodies: our digestion, breathing, temperature control and sexual function.

The nervous system controls every aspect of your life, ranging from the involuntary functions like breathing to the voluntary functions of moving. The brain, of course, is the great computer of the body where all the information from sensory nerves is transmitted and where thoughts and decisions are made, and it is from there that nerve impulses are transmitted down motor nerves to make muscles move.

Neuropathy

This is the term we use to describe nerve disease. Diabetic neuropathy is, therefore, neuropathy that occurs as a complication of a person's diabetes. It can occur in both Types 1 and Type 2 diabetes. The mechanism of nerve damage was outlined earlier in this chapter (see page 129).

The severity of symptoms that are associated with neuropathy do seem to relate to blood-glucose control. If someone with a neuropathy has his or her blood-glucose brought down to the normal level, then the symptoms of the neuropathy will often improve and may even completely reverse.

In general, diabetic neuropathy is more common:

- over the age of 40.
- in smokers of any type of tobacco: cigarettes, pipes, cigars and including marijuana.
- with higher alcohol consumption.
- in diabetics with evidence of retinopathy or nephropathy.
- when there is a history of hypertension.
- where there is evidence of cardiovascular disease.
- in taller people, who have longer nerves and therefore have more potential for nerve damage.

KEY POINTS

- About 60 per cent of diabetics have some abnormality of the nervous system.
- Complications involving the nervous system are commoner the longer the disease has been present.
- Neuropathy may be present at diagnosis of Type 2 diabetes, since the condition may have been undiagnosed for years beforehand.
- Diabetic neuropathy is most common in diabetics with poor blood-glucose control and who smoke.
- It generally takes about ten years of raised blood-glucose to cause diabetic neuropathy.

Types of neuropathy

All types of nerves can be affected, so there are several well-recognised diabetic neuropathy patterns.

Chronic peripheral neuropathy

This is also called chronic sensorimotor neuropathy. It means that it is a neuropathy that affects both motor function (nerves to muscles that operate our movements) and sensory function (nerves that supply information about touch, pain, temperature, position of joints sense and vibration sense).

Chronic peripheral neuropathy tends to take a long time to develop, without the person experiencing symptoms. It is the most common type of diabetic neuropathy. It tends to produce a glove and stocking distribution of altered touch, temperature and joint position sense. That means that the skin over the feet and lower legs, encompassing the area covered by stockings or socks, would have this numbness. It tends to be on both sides of the body. The hands can also be affected in the area that a glove would cover. However, the legs are more often affected than the arms; the hands only tend to be affected in severe neuropathy.

On physical examination the reflexes at the ankles are usually absent. Later on the reflexes at the knees are also lost. The motor component will tend to cause weakness of the muscles in those areas and the muscles may become wasted. The motor aspect tends to come later than the sensory component.

This type of neuropathy can lead to some of the problems of the diabetic foot, which we shall look at soon. It can be hard to reverse, but may improve with good diabetes control.

Acute peripheral neuritis

This is also called acute painful neuropathy, and is not very common. It tends to come on rapidly, but the good news is that whereas chronic peripheral neuropathy may not resolve, this type will often settle once good control of blood-glucose is achieved.

Pain is the main symptom. It can affect temperature sensation as well, so that the person experiences a painful, burning foot or feet. This may be especially at night when the person is trying to get to sleep. Examination may not show any abnormality. In particular, the reflexes will all be normal.

Proximal motor neuropathy

This is also called diabetic amyopathy, or Bruns-Garland's syndrome. As its name suggests, this affects motor nerves. Its main symptom is pain and paraesthesia (pins and needles) in the buttocks, hips and upper legs, with weakness and muscle wasting of the buttocks and thighs. There is often rapid and dramatic weight loss, so that the skin may sag in those areas, reflecting the loss of muscle bulk. It is most common in the middle-aged and elderly. It can begin after a time when diabetic control has been poor, perhaps after another illness.

If control can be re-established and the blood-glucose brought back to normal, then there may be gradual improvement. In order to achieve this, physiotherapy will be needed and the medical treatment may require the patient go on insulin.

Mononeuropathy

This is neuropathy affecting only one nerve. Commonly, these are the nerves that are often involved in so-called 'entrapment syndromes', meaning that a nerve is being compressed by surrounding tissues.

- The cranial nerves can be affected, so that one of the nerves to the muscles that control the movements of the eyes is affected. This can result in a lazy eye or a drooping eye. These nerves are the oculomotor nerve, usually indicated in Roman numerals as cranial nerve III; the trochlear nerve, cranial nerve IV; and the abducent nerve, cranial nerve VI.
- The median nerve at the wrist, associated with carpal tunnel syndrome, which causes pain and pins and needles in the thumb, forefinger and middle finger. It usually only affects one hand.
- The sciatic nerve, causing pain down the leg; it usually only affects one leg.
- The lateral popliteal nerve at the knee, causing foot drop; it usually only affects one side.
- The intercostal nerves that cause pains between the ribs.

Sometimes more than one nerve is involved, when the condition is called mononeuritis multiplex.

Autonomic neuropathy

The autonomic nervous system has two components, as I mentioned earlier in this chapter. The sympathetic and parasympathetic nervous systems basically carry out many of the involuntary activities of the body, meaning those that are essential, but which are carried out without you having to think about them.

Autonomic neuropathy does not tend to occur until diabetes has been present for many years. Overall, however, about 40 per cent of diabetics will have some form of autonomic neuropathy.

The following organs and systems can be affected by diabetic autonomic neuropathy.

- Eye accommodation – the muscles that move the lenses of the eyes to focus on objects may be affected, because the autonomic nerves that supply them are affected. As a result the pupils of the eyes may be reduced. In darkness they will not open up sufficiently and will cause problems seeing at night.
- Heart rhythm – the autonomic nervous system controls heartbeat rhythm. Neuropathy may result in abnormal heart rhythms, usually experienced as palpitations. Alternatively, neuropathy may prevent the heart rate from quickening up when it is needed on exertion, so the person may feel light-headed when they do too much.
- Blood pressure – the normal control of blood pressure may be lost. This can cause blood pressure drops when standing up, so that faintness can occur.
- Bladder control – the sensitivity of the bladder may be lost, so that it is not obvious when it is full and needs emptying. There may be dribbling or occasional accidents when it voids unexpectedly. The bladder may not empty completely, so there may be stagnation of urine, the ideal circumstances for a urinary infection to develop.
- Skin and perspiration – the normal heat regulation ability may be lost so that excessive perspiration occurs.
- Stomach and intestines – there may be nausea, heartburn, bloating and altered bowel patterns. The commonest symptom is constipation, although many people experience diarrhoea that is very variable and often unpredictable.
- Gall bladder – this may not empty as it should, which results in the concentration of bile and the development of gallstones.

- Sexual problems – there can be a reduction in libido and in men there may be erectile dysfunction.

As mentioned earlier, good blood-glucose control will reduce the risk and the severity of any of these complications.

Recent research suggests that statins used to reduce cholesterol levels may also be helpful in reducing nerve damage and retinopathy in diabetics.[16] A team in Denmark studied over 60,000 people with diabetes, all of whom were over the age of 40 years at diagnosis. They compared the outcomes of 15,500 patients who were on statins with 47,000 who were not taking the drugs. They found that after an average follow up time of 2.7 years, people on statins were 34 per cent less likely to be diagnosed with diabetic neuropathy. In addition, they found that they were also 40 per cent less likely to develop diabetic retinopathy.

Foot problems

The feet and the lower legs can develop complications from diabetes. As with the other complications of diabetes these can come about because of nerve damage or neuropathy and hardening of the arteries, in this case causing peripheral artery disease.

There are many things that can develop and deteriorate to affect the feet in patients with Type 2 diabetes, so it is highly important that they should always take good care of their feet. Even minor problems can worsen dramatically so constant vigilance is required.

SENSORY NEUROPATHY AND THE FOOT

- A diabetic patient with sensory neuropathy may not feel pain, heat or cold. This can be problematic, because if a cut or sore is not felt it can get worse and become infected.
- The foot muscles may not function properly and become damaged.
- The foot may become badly aligned causing too much pressure being created on one area of the foot.
- Ten per cent of diabetics will develop a foot ulcer.

PERIPHERAL ARTERY DISEASE AND THE FOOT

- Poor blood flow to the feet may result in poor or reduced healing.
- Poor blood supply means less infection-fighting white blood cells reach areas of skin that get cracked or cut, so infections are more common and healing is slowed.
- Reduced blood supply can lead to foot ulceration.
- Extreme reduction in blood supply to the tissues can result in gangrene.

Common foot problems in diabetes

Athlete's foot

This is a fungal infection of the skin, usually between the toes but sometimes on the sole of the foot. Its medical name is tinea pedis. There are several fungi that cause it including *Epidermophyton floccosum* or *Trichophyton rubrum*. They cause intense itching, redness and cracking of the skin. It is picked up in communal areas like showers and bathrooms.

The problem is that the cracking of the skin can allow other bacterial infections, which we call secondary infections, to develop. They are much more serious and can enter the body.

Athlete's foot is usually easily treated with topical cream from your doctor.

Fungal nail infections

These are quite common and produce discolouration, thickening and brittleness of the nails. The end of the nail can sometimes have a honeycomb appearance. The nails may crumble because they are so brittle.

The medical name for this is onychomycosis. It is usually caused by the same sorts of fungi that cause athlete's foot. Fungal nail infections are most likely to occur if the feet are hot and sweaty as a result of wearing shoes that are too tight and which promote perspiration.

They can be treated with anti-fungal nail paint or anti-fungal tablets. The treatment can take many weeks or months. It is better to prevent the condition with good foot care, changing socks regularly and wearing good shoes. It is a good idea to vary shoes rather than wearing the same ones every day.

Corns

These are build-ups of dried skin over bony parts of the toes or between the toes. If you develop these, it is best to have a podiatrist treat them rather than attempting to do so yourself. Infection is liable to occur with self-treatment.

Callosities

A callus (plural, callosities) is the name given to a build-up of hard skin on the underside of the foot. It can be the result of the way your feet are bearing your weight. It can also occur if you wear ill-fitting footwear or if you have an underlying skin condition.

It is part of good foot care to prevent callosities, so after a shower or bath use a pumice stone to smooth hard skin away. If they develop, then do not try to trim away with sharp objects, but allow a podiatrist to treat them.

Warts

A verruca is the correct name for a wart on the foot. It can appear singly or as clusters, usually on the soles of the feet, but also around the toes. In the early stages it is just a small, dark dot, but may become bumpy like a miniature cauliflower. When there are large clusters of them they may look like a rough callous. Verrucae are picked up from warm, moist environments, like swimming pool and sports changing rooms and showers.

If you are diabetic you should not try to treat them yourself, but allow your GP or podiatrist to deal with them. This can be done with:

- creams containing salicylic acid, which works in 75 per cent of cases.
- cryotherapy, involving freezing them with liquid nitrogen or nitrous oxide gas. This may need to be done every two to three weeks for a few months if they are extensive.
- electrosurgery, which is done under a local anaesthetic. An electric needle is inserted into the wart to boil the wart, which can then be scooped out.

- excision surgery, where the wart is cut off with a scalpel.
- laser surgery, using a laser to destroy large verrucae.

BACTERIAL INFECTIONS

The most common organisms that cause problems with foot infections of cracks and diabetic ulcers are *Staphylococcus aureus, Streptococcus pyogenes* and various *Bacteroides*. The latter grow well when there is little oxygen so they thrive when the tissues are relatively poorly supplied with oxygen-rich blood. This is common in diabetes, which makes good foot care all the more important.

General dryness of the skin

As a result of poor blood supply or neuropathy, the skin texture can change so that it becomes less elastic and dry. This can predispose to cracking of the skin and the risk of bacteria entering the cracks to produce an infection. The development of a skin ulcer is also more likely. It is sensible to keep the skin as supple as possible by applying a skin moisturiser every day as part of general skin care.

Ingrowing toenail

This occurs when the nail edges grow into the skin. The skin then swells, gets cut by the nail edge and often becomes infected.

To prevent an ingrowing toenail, look after the nails and keep them cut regularly. The correct way to cut the nails is straight across, rather than cutting down to try and shape them. This shaping tends to cause sharp edges to appear that can traumatise the skin, which swells and the ingrowing tendency develops. This is most likely to happen as the nails get thicker, which occurs as one ages. It is also more probable if a fungal nail infection occurs as well.

Ulcers

A diabetic foot ulcer occurs when part of the skin breaks down to expose the underlying tissue. If you have diabetes this can develop after relatively little skin trauma. If you stub your foot or scratch it, the skin may not heal as well as it would in a person without diabetes. The danger is that the ulcer can enlarge, becoming more extensive to expose underlying structures in the foot.

As with most of the skin complications discussed in this chapter, an ulcer is more likely because of neuropathy, when the foot becomes less sensitive, and when the blood supply becomes poor. This is why it is very important for diabetics to check their feet every day, because diminished sensation may make them more prone to ulceration.

Ulcers commonly become infected, which makes them harder to heal. There is then the danger of the infection spreading to the blood and a serious infection called septicaemia being the result. Generally, however, ulcers can be treated with good nursing care. The main thing is to try to prevent them.

KEY POINT

About 25 per cent of diabetic admissions to hospital are because of foot ulcers.

Gangrene

This is the worst-case scenario with the diabetic foot. It occurs because of the poor blood supply to the extremities. Thus, ulcers in the toes, which are extremities, can occur.

Gangrenous tissue goes black and becomes very friable. There can be great pain, or paradoxically, there can be remarkably little pain if there is also neuropathy that causes numbness.

The treatment may involve surgery to remove dead skin that sloughs off. This is to allow healing from underneath. Other surgical procedures that might help are bypass surgery by a vascular surgeon, where he or she may graft a vein from another part of the body to the ischaemic part of the foot to improve blood supply. Another procedure is a balloon angioplasty, which involves inserting a tiny catheter into an artery and inflating a miniature balloon to enlarge a blocked vessel. A stent, a miniature wire cylinder may be left in the vessel to hold it open to maintain blood flow.

Gangrene can slowly spread, which is more likely the higher the blood-glucose levels. It may be necessary to amputate a foot or even part of a leg. This is only done in the extreme case in order to protect the tissues further up the limb.

Changing shape of the foot

Over a long period of time the shape of the foot may change. Neuropathy can cause weakness of the foot muscles so that the instep, which is a natural arch caused by the pull of muscles, may collapse. This then alters the whole anatomy of the foot. As a result, the way that the foot bears weight changes predisposing to some of the complications considered above.

A bunion can develop. The medical name for this is hallux valgus, which means that the big toe (hallux) deviates inwards (valgus). A bunionette may also occur, referring to the same thing happening with the little toe, pushing it inwards as well.

Hammer toes also occur, whereby the inner toes become bunched up and clawed. One toe can even get pushed under another.

This can all result in the development of a Charcot foot, in which the foot becomes totally misshapen. It was first described by the famous French neurologist Jean-Martin Charcot (1825–1893). As the result of a neuropathy causing numbness and loss of the ability to sense the position of the foot, the muscles lose their ability to support the joints in the foot properly. The numbness allows minor traumas such as sprains and stress fractures to go undetected and untreated, leading to ligament slackness, small joint dislocations, bone erosion, cartilage damage and deformity of the foot.

The bones most often affected in a Charcot foot are the metatarsals and the tarsals, located in the forefoot and mid foot. It is also more likely to occur the more overweight the person becomes. Many people with Type 2 diabetes are overweight.

It is most likely to develop 10–15 years after the diagnosis of diabetes. Orthotic advice from the podiatrist is needed, but surgical correction may be necessary either by a podiatric surgeon or an orthopaedic surgeon.

TIPS FOR GOOD FOOT CARE

- Check your feet every night and morning for blisters, sores, ulcers, athlete's foot and other infections, indicated by redness.
- Maintain good control of the diabetes, since foot problems are likelier to occur if the blood-glucose is out of control.

- Do not smoke, since this worsens arteriosclerosis and reduces blood flow.
- Wash your feet in warm water with a mild soap. Always test the water before washing by dipping an elbow in it because neuropathy may have damaged temperature sensation and you may not feel hot water with your feet. Do not soak the feet, just wash them, because the skin can get crinkly and can crack, which can allow infection in. Dry well, especially between the toes.
- Apply moisturiser cream if the skin is dry.
- Gently smooth corns and callosities with a pumice stone or an emery board. This is best done after washing which will soften the skin.
- Check toenails every week. Always trim them with a nail clipper, going straight across, not shaping them or cutting too short.
- Always wear well-fitting shoes or slippers with a closed toe. Avoid sandals, which expose the toes to trauma.
- Always wear socks or stockings.
- When choosing new shoes, go for a fitting in the middle of the day. The feet swell as the day goes on and shoes measured early in the day may be too tight later on.
- Choose flat-soled shoes rather than high heels, since high-heeled shoes will tend to cause bunching of the toes and throw pressure onto the front of the foot.
- Avoid warming your feet in front of fires.
- At first sight of any problem, consult your doctor.
- Have an annual check up by your doctor. Make sure that you are tested for nerve damage.
- See your podiatrist every three months.

Skin problems

It is not just the skin of the legs and the feet that is affected in diabetes. The skin anywhere on the body can be prone to complications.

The sort of problems that can occur include:

- dry, itchy skin.
- bacterial infections, spots, pimples and abscesses.
- folliculitis, producinvg small red inflammatory spots around the hair follicles.
- styes in the eyes.
- blisters, because the skin can become dry and less elastic it is more susceptible to shearing forces when walking.
- infections around nails of hands, known as paronychia.
- pigmentation changes, causing darkened skin in armpits and groin.

The skin can also be subject to pain; this is the neuropathic pain referred to in the section on neuropathy.

ACANTHOSIS NIGRICANS

This is a condition that can occur ahead of the diagnosis of Type 2 diabetes. It is a pigmentary condition affecting the areas round the neck, the armpits and the groin, which may all seem to become darker. The skin may also become harder and may be prone to secondary infections. It may be more likely to produce body odour.

It is more commonly observed in people of Afro-Caribbean or Hispanic origin.

It can occur in other conditions, such as hypothyroidism, cancer and obesity.

Mouth disorders

Medically, we refer to periodontal disease, meaning disease of the bones and the gum tissues that hold the teeth in place.

Gum disease can affect one in three people with diabetes. The problems occur because of the affect that long-term high blood-glucose has on blood vessels and their supply of blood to the tissues. The blood supply to the bones of the jaws can weaken them and the overlying gums, making them more liable to infection.

Periodontal disease can cause the following:

- bleeding gums, even from gentle brushing or flossing.
- swollen, red or tender gums – this is called gingivitis.
- gum recession.
- increasing plaque on the teeth.
- loose teeth – often because of disease of the gums.
- presence of pus between teeth and the gums – this is called pyorrhoea.
- persistent bad breath – called halitosis.
- mouth infections, including gum boils and thrush (seen as white or yellow patches in the mouth). Apart from the increased

susceptibility to infections this may come about because there may be higher amounts of glucose in the mouth, which allows microorganisms to thrive.

Gum disease directly correlates with blood-glucose control, so the better the control of the diabetes the lower the risk of developing gum disease.

It is important to maintain good dental hygiene with regular brushing and flossing. Also, see your dentist and dental hygienist at least twice a year to ensure that gum disease does not develop or progress.

Smoking increases the risk of periodontal disease so it is worth stopping or avoiding the habit.

Bladder and urinary problems

Diabetes predisposes people to all types of infections. Urinary tract infections, typically producing cystitis, are the most common ones. The symptoms of a urinary infection are abdominal cramps, increased frequency of passage of urine, difficulty or pain on passing urine and blood in the urine. The urine may be malodorous. The presence of any of these symptoms should prompt a visit to the doctor and investigation by testing a sample of urine. The symptoms should never be ignored, because they could be due to other pathology, including urinary tract cancer. The higher the blood-glucose, the more likely urinary infections are to occur. It is important to have these treated with antibiotics if confirmed in order to prevent an infection ascending upwards through the urinary tract to affect the kidneys.

Pelvic floor exercises might help

These are often known as Kegel exercises. They were first developed by a gynaecologist for use by women after childbirth to regain tone.

They are useful if you have:

- stress incontinence – leaking urine when you laugh, cough, sneeze, jog, or lift something heavy.
- urge incontinence – a need to urinate that is so strong you can't reach the toilet in time.
- erectile dysfunction (see below).

How to do Kegel exercises for women

Kegels are easy to do and can be done anywhere without anyone knowing.

Your aim is to discover and be aware of the muscles you use to stop urinating. Squeeze these muscles for three seconds and then relax for three seconds. Your stomach and thigh muscles should not tighten when you do this.

Add one second each week until you are able to squeeze for ten seconds and relax for ten seconds each time.

Repeat this exercise 10–15 times per session. Try to do this at least three times a day.

Sexual problems

There can be a variety of problems for both sexes.

Reduced libido

The sex drive can be affected in both men and women. This can come about through psychological reasons, for example as a result of having been given the diagnosis of diabetes. Some people react adversely to this and feel that it in some way diminishes him or her as a person. This is not the case at all, but the erroneous thought may need to be dealt with, possibly by counselling.

Reduced libido can also be the result of physical complications from the diabetes, as a result of damage to nerves and to hardening of arteries.

All of the following factors can affect libido.

- Relationship problems
- Physical diabetic complications – neuropathy and hardening of arteries
- Reduced sex hormone levels
- Impending menopause
- Stress
- Tiredness
- Depression
- Over-consumption of alcohol
- An underactive thyroid (hypothyroidism)
- Some drugs, such as beta blockers for hypertension.

If you experience diminished libido, consult your GP who can do tests. These may reveal a physical cause that medication or adjustment of medication can improve, or counselling may be available.

In general, good control of the diabetes will often help. You can also try some self-help techniques, which we will look at in the section on sexual problems in Chapter 10 (*Using the Life Cycle with Type 2 diabetes*).

Reduced ability to achieve orgasm

This can occur as a result of psychological factors or physical ones. In general, mutual discussion between partners can help to remove anxiety. If you can agree that achieving an orgasm may not be the most important aspect of lovemaking, then you will immediately reduce anxiety about it. Being patient and being gentle and caring, enjoying caressing, foreplay and loving may make the whole act more mutually satisfying.

Erectile dysfunction

This is a problem that affects about 75 per cent of all men at some point in their lives, so it is not necessarily a diabetes-related problem. Erectile dysfunction does, however, affect 35–75 per cent of male diabetics.

It usually takes the form of difficulty in achieving or maintaining an erection. Sexual penetration may be difficult or prove impossible because the penis does not get a sufficiently firm erection.

The cause is hard to pinpoint, but is probably a mixture of nerve damage and hardening of the arteries. Anxiety often plays a large part in this. We will return to this in Chapter 10 (*Using the Life Cycle with Type 2 diabetes*) since there are strategies that can be used to overcome it.

Good diabetic control, increased exercise and weight reduction may all help as well. Pelvic floor exercises have also been found to have some effect. A study from the University of Bristol in the UK in 2005 found that pelvic exercises helped 40 per cent of men with erectile dysfunction regain normal erectile function. An additional 33.5 per cent significantly improved erectile function.[17]

Kegel exercises for men

Halfway through urination, try to stop or slow the flow of urine. Do not tense the muscles in your buttocks, legs or abdomen and do not hold your breath. When you can slow or stop the flow of urine, you have successfully located the muscles that help to control the passing of urine.

Once you have located the muscles and know what they feel like, then try these Kegel exercises for men:

- Contract these muscles for a slow count of five.
- Release the muscles to a slow count of five.
- Repeat ten times.
- Do a set of ten Kegels, three times a day.

Medical treatment for erectile dysfunction

Your GP can prescribe the following drugs, which are very effective in achieving an erection: Viagra, Cialis and Levitra.

It is also possible to use another drug called alprostadil, a type of prostaglandin. This can be used as:

- a gel that is rubbed on the glans penis, the head of the penis.

- a pellet that is inserted into the urethra, the penis tube.
- an intracavernosal injection into the base of the penis.

Other methods include:

- a rubber ring that is placed around the base of the penis to keep it erect.
- a vacuum pump (battery- or hand-operated) creates a vacuum that causes the penis to fill up with blood and become erect.

Female sexual dysfunction

Libido can be affected, but neuropathy can also affect the genitals to reduce sensation, or on the contrary, to make the genitals so sensitive that the person experiences pain. This may make the person want to avoid sex entirely. Diabetes can also affect the female sex hormones, resulting in dryness and lack of vaginal lubrication. Discussion with your GP may yield a solution, such as prescribing creams to help lubrication or hormonal pessaries.

In women who wish to become pregnant, sexual dysfunction is not in itself a barrier to becoming pregnant. It may also help to know that there will be no reduction in fertility.

Stomach and bowel problems

The stomach and small and large intestines may all be affected in Type 2 diabetes as a result of diminished blood supply to them and from nerve damage in the form of autonomic neuropathy. This may affect the vagus nerve, which is cranial nerve X.

The way that the stomach and the intestines contract to move food and digested products along may be affected. This can be an over-contraction or an under-contraction that may result in abdominal pains, nausea, bloating or either constipation or increased looseness of the bowel habit.

Undigested food may actually cause a blockage and an infection can result from stagnation. This is called gastroparesis, which may result in uneven absorption of carbohydrates. This can have a compounding effect on blood-glucose control since food and nutrients may be absorbed at different rates, not always predictably.

The treatment is:

- Good control of the diabetes.
- Dietary manipulation, possibly including portion control and timing of meals, so that you eat small and often, perhaps up to six times a day.
- Drugs that may help:
    - metoclopramide, which increases muscle contractions in the upper digestive tract
    - the antibiotic, erythromycin
    - anti-nausea drugs, such as domperidone.

Psychological complications

These vary from sleep disturbance to anxiety and depression. We will consider these more fully in Chapter 10 (*Using the Life Cycle with Type 2 diabetes*).

Chapter 8

Lifestyle changes to treat Type 2 diabetes

The sort of lifestyle changes that we are going to cover in this chapter are sensible ones that doctors advise everyone to consider, not just people with diabetes. They are changes that will result in better health for anyone. In people with Type 2 diabetes, they may be sufficient in themselves to control the diabetes and prevent complications, without the necessity of taking medication. Even if medication is needed, then a good diet will help the medication to work more effectively.

Lifestyle changes recommended in the treatment of Type 2 diabetes:

- Diet modification
- Weight control
- Adequate exercise.

Diet and nutrition

The word diet does not mean something that you do in order to reduce weight; it merely means the food that you normally eat. Everyone has a diet, but this is not the same as being 'on a diet'.

In Type 2 diabetes it is important to ensure that you have a healthy and balanced diet. As much as you can, you should eat unprocessed foods.

A dietician may help

Some people with diabetes may have special dietary needs, so it is up to your GP to assess this. If necessary, a referral may be made to a dietician in order to tailor a diet to you. This is more likely if you:

- are overweight or obese – a weight-reducing diet is needed that still maintains diabetic control.
- have central obesity – you need to take measures to reduce abdominal fat.
- have high blood pressure – salt may need restricting in your diet.
- have kidney complications – proteins may need to be restricted.
- are vegetarian – to ensure you are achieving the right balance of proteins, carbohydrates and fats.
- are on medication – some drugs prescribed for Type 2 diabetes, such as sulphonylureas and thiazolidinediones, can make some people put on weight.

KEY POINT

Eighty per cent of Type 2 diabetics in the UK are overweight and need to reduce weight.

Eat regular meals

If you want to achieve a regular level of blood-glucose then it makes sense to eat regularly so that your body gets used to regular food at regular intervals and deals with it most effectively. If you sometimes miss breakfast, skip lunch and tend to snatch food when the opportunity arises, then you have some degree of dietary chaos and the blood-glucose will reflect that. A rule of thumb to use is to eat at four-hour intervals.

Start the day with a healthy breakfast

Having a good breakfast is probably one of the best things that you can do to help your health. There seems to be truth in the old adage that you should breakfast like a king, lunch like a prince and dine like a pauper. A healthy breakfast is good for the heart, cholesterol levels and may even reduce the risk of developing diabetes.

Research from Boston, USA, supports the concept that breakfast is the most important meal of the day. It has been found that the rate of obesity, high blood pressure and insulin resistance was 35–50 per cent lower in those who had breakfast compared to those who miss it. In addition, those who miss breakfast seem more likely to have problems with their cholesterol.

The researchers suspect that breakfast stimulates your natural insulin and primes the body's metabolism to control blood-sugar levels, which are of course related to how hungry or energetic one feels. By not having that stimulation, the body could ultimately develop some resistance to the insulin, and that can be when problems start.

GLYCAEMIC INDEX (GI)

This puts foods on a scale according to the rate at which they are broken down to form glucose. Foods are given a score out of 100. Foods are only given a GI score if they contain carbohydrates.

High glycaemic index foods are broken down rapidly into glucose.

FOOD	GI
High glycaemic index foods have a GI of 70 or more. For example:	
White rice	98
Cornflakes	85
French fries	75
White bread	70

Medium glycaemic index foods have a GI of 56–69. For example:	
Rye bread	65
Cheese and tomato pizza	60
Digestive biscuits	59
Pitta bread	57
Sultanas	56

Low glycaemic index foods are broken down slowly to produce glucose. They have a GI of 55 or less. Thus, the following are low-GI foods:	
Sweetcorn	55
Banana	55
Wholemeal bread	53
Baked beans	48
Apples	38
Low-fat yoghurt	14

The higher the glycaemic index of a food, the quicker it will raise blood-glucose. The lower the glycaemic index, the slower the absorption of carbohydrates and the easier it will be to control blood-glucose.

Low glycaemic index diet

In the UK the NHS recommends that Type 2 diabetics should follow a low-GI diet, as opposed to a low-carbohydrate diet, which used to be the recommendation. The low-GI diet works best when portions are kept under control, so it is usually a case of developing discipline and self-control, avoiding second helpings and getting out of the 'eating-up' habit, whereby you finish all the food at a meal, despite having had your requirements.

Know the food groups and balance them

Spending some time to learn about the different types of food is a good place to begin.

There are five main food groups.

- Starchy foods – for example: bread, rice, pasta and potatoes
- Fruit and vegetables
- Milk and dairy foods and alternatives to dairy products
- Protein foods – meat, fish, eggs, nuts, beans and pulses
- Fatty and sugary foods.

Starchy foods

Choose carbohydrate foods with a low GI but which also have a high fibre content. For example: bread, rice, potatoes and pasta.

Rule of thumb: make starchy foods one third of every meal.

Fruit and vegetables

These are packed with vitamins, minerals and fibre, but are low in fat and calories. These are good for general health.

Rule of thumb: make fruit and vegetables up to half of every meal and have at least five portions a day. A portion is equal to a handful.

Milk and dairy products

Milk, cheese and yoghurt are rich in calcium and are good for teeth and bones. They are a good source of protein.

Alternatives to dairy foods are prepared from plants sources, like soya, almonds, cashews and coconut. Lactose-free dairy products are made from cow's milk, but prepared in a way to reduce the lactose content for people with lactose intolerance.

Rule of thumb: have three portions a day. For example, an eight-ounce glass – one cup or 230 millilitres – of milk or a dairy alternative such as soya or almond milk is one portion.

Protein foods

These are rich in protein and are needed to build muscle cells. They also contain minerals, like iron, and essential vitamins. Oily fish is rich in omega oils, which are beneficial to the heart.

Rule of thumb – these should take up a third of your diet. Have two to three portions a day. One egg is a portion, as is a serving of fish or meat that is about the size of a deck of cards.

Fatty and sugary foods

You do not have to avoid these totally, but they should be restricted. You can still have cake or biscuits as occasional treats.

Rule of thumb – only allow one portion (two biscuits) a day.

Increase your fibre and reduce the fat

Increasing the amount of fibre you eat and reducing your fat intake, especially saturated fat (see *A short lesson about fats and oils*, page 166) can help manage your cholesterol and will help control diabetes.

The following tips may help.

- Increase the intake of high-fibre foods, such as wholegrain bread, cereals, beans, lentils, fruit and vegetables.
- Choose foods that are low in fat – try replacing butter, ghee and coconut oil with low-fat spreads and vegetable oil.
- Use skimmed and semi-skimmed milk. Alternatives include lactose- and casein-free milk and soya, rice, oat, almond or coconut milk.
- Use low-fat yoghurts or alternatives like soya or coconut milk yoghurts. (See *A yoghurt a day may keep Type 2 diabetes away*, page 171.)

- Eat fish and lean meat rather than fatty or processed meat, such as bacon, sausages and burgers.
- Grill, bake, poach or steam food instead of frying or roasting it.
- Avoid high-fat foods, such as mayonnaise, chips, crisps, pasties, poppadoms and samosas.

Food labelling

It is worth getting into the habit of checking food labelling. In the UK there are two basic types of food labelling:

- Daily amount guidelines
- Traffic light system.

The daily amount guideline will quantify the amounts of fats, carbohydrates, proteins and salt, and provide a calorie content per 100-gram and per serving. The amounts will then be compared against recommended daily intake of those foods.

The traffic light system is easy to use. Foods are colour coded red, amber and green like a traffic signal to indicate the levels of the various components in the product you are buying.

- Red = high level, so you should choose this food less often.
- Amber = medium level, so you can choose this food more often than red, but less than green.
- Green = low level, so eat this food as often as you wish.

My suggestion is that in diabetes you want to avoid or only have as a special treat those foods labelled red for their high sugar or carbohydrate content. The traffic light system is easier to follow than the daily amount guidelines.

Eat the colours of the rainbow when looking at fruit and vegetables

As mentioned above, you should be trying to have five portions of fruit and vegetables a day. In addition, by varying the colours that you eat, you can get even more benefit and get the widest range of healthy nutrients. All you have to do is use the rainbow as a guide.

Red fruit and vegetables

These are good sources of lycopene, ellagic acid and quercetin. Tomatoes are rich in lycopene, which is known to be beneficial for men and prostate health and is also protective to the heart. Ellagic acid is abundant in raspberries, strawberries and pomegranates. It is a powerful antioxidant that seems to have anti-cancer properties, and is especially protective to the bowel. Apples are rich in quercetin, another antioxidant, which helps the body deal with allergens. Recently it has been found to help asthma.

These foods are also rich in iridoids, which can lower advanced glycation end products (AGEs), which we will consider in *Understanding AGEs and your diet*, page 168

Yellow and orange fruit and vegetables

These contain beta-carotene, flavonoids and lycopene. Beta-carotene is converted into vitamin A by the liver. It is good for eye health and has a beneficial effect on eyesight. In addition, it has been shown to decrease cholesterol levels in the liver. Think of adding apricots, oranges, lemons, peaches, papayas and pineapples to your weekly fruit shopping, along with sweetcorn, peppers and butternut squashes.

Green fruit and vegetables

These are packed with goodness. They contain iron, carotenoids (which protect the eyes) and vitamins C and E. The nutrients found in these vegetables reduce cancer risks, lower blood pressure and LDL cholesterol levels, help the function of the digestive tract, support retinal health and vision and boost the immune system.

Blue and purple fruit and vegetables

These include prunes, grapes and raisins, all of which are rich in flavonoids, which boost the immune system and are anti-inflammatory. Blueberries are particularly rich in lutein. It has been shown to be good for eye health, especially in the middle-aged and elderly. In addition, it is beneficial for the heart. Aubergines are rich in B vitamins, plus potassium, iron and zinc, and are another good one for prostate health. About a third of a large aubergine would count as a portion.

Blue and purple produce are also rich in iridoids that can lower advanced glycation end products, AGEs, which we shall consider on page 168.

White fruit and vegetables

These contain nutrients such as beta-glucans and lignans that boost the immune system. They activate natural killer B and T cells, which are thought to reduce the risk of colon, breast and prostate cancer. There is some evidence that they also help to balance hormone levels, reducing the risk of hormone-related cancers. Here you can think of bananas, pears, white nectarines, garlic, onions, cauliflowers and mushrooms.

Potatoes are pretty much a mainstay of the British diet, but unfortunately they do not count towards your five a day. Nor do yams or cassavas, because they are all starchy foods. So, it is a good thing to get in the habit of making vegetables a bigger part of a meal, as we will consider when we come to portion control later in this chapter. Vegetables should not be thought of as just a little something to add to the plate beside the meat and potatoes.

The DESMOND programme

This is a programme, which I mentioned in Chapter 6 (*How diabetes is diagnosed and managed*). DESMOND stands for Diabetes Education and Self Management for Ongoing and Newly Diagnosed. It specialises in helping people with Type 2 diabetes to self-manage their condition effectively. This programme is recommended by the National Institute for Health and Clinical Excellence (NICE).

It is a six-hour programme, presented over one or two days. Up to ten people with Type 2 diabetes or with pre-diabetes meet with two trained DESMOND healthcare professionals or educators. It is available as a Newly Diagnosed Module (for those within the first 12 months of diagnosis) or as Foundation Modules (for those with established diabetes).

Course attendees can be accompanied by a person of their choice. The aim is to provide a working understanding of the condition and give advice and strategies to sustain the person's motivation.

Contents of the DESMOND programme

- Thoughts and feelings of the participants about diabetes.
- Understanding diabetes and glucose: what happens in the body.

- Understanding the risk factors and complications associated with diabetes.
- Understanding more about monitoring and medication.
- How to take control: food choices and physical activity.
- Planning for the future.

The beauty of the course is in helping people to understand the condition. In part this is done by dispelling many of the myths about the condition and by offering practical advice about how it can affect your health currently and in the future.

The Mediterranean diet

There has been a great deal of interest in the Mediterranean diet and its benefit in Type 2 diabetes. Basically, it is a non-restrictive diet, meaning that there is no calorie reduction or portion reduction; it is an alteration of the types of foods that you eat.

The PREDIMED-Reus nutrition intervention randomised trial[18] has shown that the incidence of diabetes in people eating the Mediterranean diet supplemented with either olive oil or nuts is significantly lower than in those people who regularly eat a non-Mediterranean diet.

A review of 19 studies that included more than 160,000 people in different countries studied over an average of 5.5 years showed that a Mediterranean diet was associated with a 21 per cent lower risk of diabetes than other diets.

The characteristics of the so-called Mediterranean diet:

- High levels of fruits and vegetables, breads and other cereals, potatoes, beans, nuts and seeds.

- Olive oil is the only oil product allowed.
- Moderate amounts of dairy products, fish and poultry, but very little red meat.
- Eggs allowed, but no more than four per week and no more than one on any day.
- Wine consumed in moderate amounts – two glasses maximum per day for men and one glass for women

The fish and the olive oil appear to be two of the most significant features of the diet. Olive oil seems to be rich in monounsaturated fatty acids. It is suggested that its benefit may be in improving the way that serotonin, the 'happiness neurotransmitter' is bound to its receptors.

Oily fish is rich in omega-3 fats, which seem to be the factors that benefit us most. They certainly seem to have an anti-inflammatory effect.

A short lesson about fats and oils

Everyone knows that you must not take too much fat into your system, and we hear much about the benefits of various types of oils. Understandably, there is a lot of confusion about fats and oils, so I shall try to present my own understanding as simply as possible.

There are three basic types of fats – saturated, monounsaturated and polyunsaturated.

Saturated fats

Saturated fats are found in animal products such as meat, eggs and dairy products. In general, these are considered 'bad' fats, since they have a tendency to push up your cholesterol and promote inflammation. They do this because arachidonic acid – one of the fatty acids found in these fats – is broken down by enzymes into prostaglandins and leukotrienes, both of which are known to trigger inflammation.

Monounsaturated fats

Monounsaturated fats are found in various nuts (including peanuts, walnuts and almonds), avocados and olive oil. They help to lower cholesterol and are 'good' fats, which means they can help to reduce inflammation.

Polyunsaturated fats

Polyunsaturated fats are the best ones, and they are found in seafood and fish, corn oil and sunflower oil. They help to lower cholesterol and they are also anti-inflammatory. They are composed of two groups of essential fatty acids, called omega-3 and omega-6. In general, omega-3s have a more anti-inflammatory effect than the omega-6s. Indeed, some omega-6s actually promote inflammation. The Mediterranean diet has a better balance between omega-3s and omega-6s than the British and other Western diets. Meat, which is high in omega-6s, is reduced in the Mediterranean diet in favour of foods high in omega-3s.

There are two types of omega-3s: those with long chains and those with short chains. The long chains are mainly found in oily fish. The two main long chain ones are called eicosapentaenoic acid (EPA) and docosahexaenoic acid (DHA). These are anti-inflammatory and they have been found to be good for both arthritis and the heart and, seemingly, also depression. Short-chain omega-3s are found in foods like soya, flax, pumpkin seeds, walnuts and leafy green vegetables. These can be converted by the body into long-chain fatty acids which do the most good.

You will find that lots of foods, like spreads, juices and even milk have added omega-3s. This is good in that the average British diet is really quite deficient in omega-3s. Yet the thing is that it is more efficient to get the omega-3s in their natural form from oily fish such as salmon, mackerel and sardines. Aim at having two or, even better, three portions a week.

Take care, though, if you are prone to gout! This is not because of the omega oils, but because of the high purine content of oily fish. When purine is broken down by the body, uric acid is produced and, if you suffer from gout, crystals of this uric acid can form in the kidneys and joints.

Oddly enough, olive oil (the only oil in the Mediterranean diet) contains no omega-3s. Its main constituent is oleic acid, which belongs to the less beneficial omega-9s. It is a bit of a mystery, but research is ongoing into the undoubted benefits of olive oil. It certainly seems to have marked anti-inflammatory effects.

Understanding AGEs and your diet

As discussed in Chapter 5 (*The reasons why complications occur*), advanced glycation end products (AGEs) are thought to be one of the reasons why damage occurs. It relates to the high levels of glucose and the increased tendency that there will be to build up AGEs.

To recap, AGEs form within the body when proteins or fats combine with sugars through the process of glycation. AGEs affect the normal functioning of cells, making them more susceptible to damage.

The body does its best to eliminate them, but if it is overwhelmed by too many the damage begins. The ageing process will bring about an accumulation of AGEs, which is thought to be one of the mechanisms that cause many chronic conditions like Alzheimer's disease and cardiovascular and liver disease.

Eating a diet rich in meat will promote more AGEs. The high protein and fat provide the building bricks, as do sugary foods and highly processed foods. Of course, having Type 2 diabetes provides the other essential building block, blood-glucose. So to reduce the effect of AGEs, the aim should be to keep blood-glucose down to the normal levels of non-diabetic people and to limit those foods that promote AGEs.

- Dry heat promotes AGEs formation by more than 10–100-fold compared to uncooked foods.
- Meats high in protein and fat are likely to form AGEs during cooking.
- Carbohydrate-rich foods such as fruits, vegetables and wholegrains maintain low AGEs levels after cooking.
- Foods cooked with moist heat, shorter cooking times and lower temperatures, and acidic ingredients such as vinegar or lemon juice produced the least amount of AGEs.

Tips to reduce AGEs

- Grilling or barbecuing food with dry heat will tend to produce AGEs. Salads are healthier because you are not cooking.
- Steaming, boiling and poaching are less likely to produce AGEs.
- You can reduce the AGEs in grilling by using an acid-based marinade containing citrus fruits or vinegar.
- Prepare foods from raw and reduce packaged snacks and ready-meals.

- The rapid browning of food – under the grill, on the barbeque or in the frying pan – indicates that you are producing AGEs. It is better to eat meats done this way rare rather than well done. It is also better to use medium heat rather than high heat and to cook for a little longer.
- Making sure that 50 per cent of your food intake is fruits and vegetables will reduce the AGEs because of their high antioxidant levels.

Foods high in AGEs

- Sugary items such as biscuits, confectionary and cakes, fizzy drinks and pastries
- Processed foods, including packaged meats and cheese
- High-fat (especially red) meats
- Fats, including butter, margarine and cooking oils
- All fried foods.

Foods low in AGEs

- Fruits and vegetables
- Seafood
- Wholegrains
- Low-fat breads
- Pasta
- Vegetarian meat substitutes.

A yoghurt a day may keep Type 2 diabetes away

Research from the University of Cambridge in the UK, which was published in 2014, suggests that a simple thing to do to prevent Type 2 diabetes is to add low-fat yoghurt to your diet.[19] This study looked at over 4,200 people. During an 11-year follow-up, about 750 people developed Type 2 diabetes. They were compared with 3,500 randomly selected people for comparison. When their diets were examined they found that those people who ate more low-fat fermented dairy products, such as yoghurt, fromage frais and low-fat cottage cheese had a 25 per cent lower risk of developing diabetes compared to those who did not eat any.

Fascinatingly, when the researchers looked specifically at yoghurt, the risk of developing diabetes was reduced by almost 30 per cent. The lowest risk was in people who ate a small pot of yoghurt four or five times a week.

Another study from Harvard University in the USA showed a similar result.[20] They analysed the dietary habits of more than 190,000 people and found a clear association between a high consumption of yoghurt and a low risk of Type 2 diabetes. They found that eating a single 28-gram pot of yoghurt a day was associated with an 18 per cent reduction in risk.

Watch out for your salt intake

The fact is that salt helps to increase blood pressure by affecting internal regulatory mechanisms that push the pressure higher. One must appreciate that blood pressure is very important. It is a real risk factor for strokes, heart failure and heart attacks. Sodium seems to be the culprit, and since salt is the main source of sodium in the diet it is the obvious thing to reduce to minimise your risk.

Adults are advised to consume no more than six grams of salt a day. That is about a teaspoon. The average intake in the UK is about nine grams, or about 50 per cent more than is recommended. For a large number of people who already have raised blood pressure that is very significant.

Be careful if you have a salt tooth and consider using oregano

It is well known that too much salt is not good for you. It is not that it can directly affect diabetes, but it can contribute to elevating blood pressure which, as we saw in Chapter 5 (*The reasons why complications occur*) can be both a cause and a consequence of arteriosclerosis and cardiovascular disease. These are potential complications of Type 2 diabetes so reducing salt can reduce the risk of a complication of diabetes.

Some people seem to have a salt tooth, just as people can have a sweet tooth that makes them crave sweets and carbs. An interesting study from Brazil looked at whether people with a salt tooth, that is a preference for saltier food, were more likely to have high blood pressure. They looked at four separate groups of people, each group consisting of 30 individuals. Two of the groups were people aged in their thirties. One group had normal blood pressure and the other had high blood pressure. They also looked at two groups aged in their seventies; one group with and one without high blood pressure.

All groups were offered three different types of French bread. Each of them contained different quantities of salt. There was a significant difference between the amounts of salt. Interestingly, none of the people in either age group with normal blood pressure showed a preference for the salty bread. Instead, the older age group preferred the medium salted bread, while the younger age group preferred the lightly salted bread. The people with high blood pressure in both age groups preferred the saltiest bread.

Two weeks later the groups were randomly offered the same three breads and salt combinations. This time, though, the breads were also flavoured with the herb, oregano. This time, all groups opted for the lightly salted bread.

The study rather implies that people who have high blood pressure have a salt tooth. It may be that this is significant in helping to produce the high blood pressure over a long time. Yet the interesting thing is that by using herbs it is possible to overcome that salt desire, or to reduce the amount that one wants to have.

It is never a bad thing to limit your salt intake. If you automatically reach for the salt cellar even before you taste your food, then you may be inadvertently taking in more salt than you need. Why not try reducing that quantity, especially if you have high blood pressure? Or, add herbs like oregano.

Alcohol

You do not have to stop drinking because you are diabetic. You should, however, limit your alcohol intake to the recommended safe limits. Indeed, a little alcohol a day seems to be beneficial in reducing the risk of coronary artery disease. Too much, on the other hand, increases the risk.

This trend can be shown in the J-shaped curve phenomenon in Figure 17. This shows the risk of death from coronary artery disease when measured against the number of alcoholic drinks consumed a day. This is highly relevant for diabetics, since arteriosclerosis and heart disease are known complications of diabetes.

The graph starts by showing that the death risk is standard when there is no alcohol in the diet. But with moderate drinking the risk drops, then it increases as the average number of daily alcohol units increases.

Figure 17: The J-shaped curve

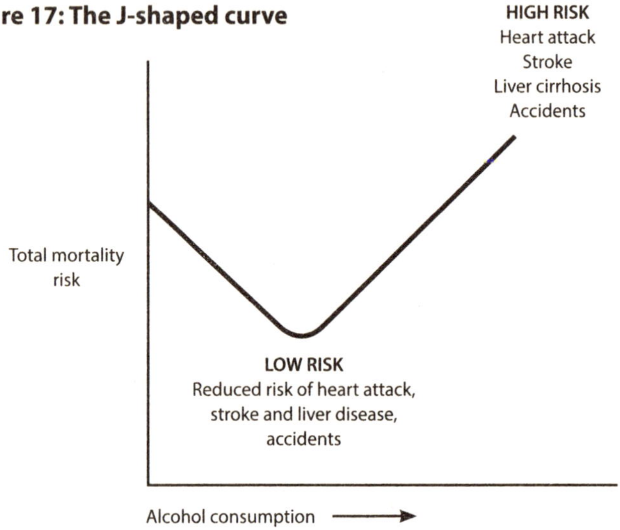

KEY POINTS

The Royal College of Physicians recommends that:

- men should not drink more than 21 units of alcohol a week.
- sensible drinking for men – the daily alcohol intake should not exceed three to four units.
- women should not drink more than 14 units a week.
- sensible drinking for women – the daily alcohol intake should not exceed two to three units.
- continued drinking at the upper limit is not advised, and at least two alcohol-free days a week should be taken.
- as a rule of thumb, heavy drinking is defined as six units in six hours.
- a unit is either a small measure of spirit, a small glass of wine or a half pint of beer or lager.

It is sensible to also only drink with meals or soon after them, especially if you are taking oral hypoglycaemic drugs, since the effect could cause the blood-glucose to drop substantially.

Portion control the plate way

Choosing how much food to eat can be confusing initially, but a useful method of portion control is the plate method. This allows you to build up a plan for your meals.

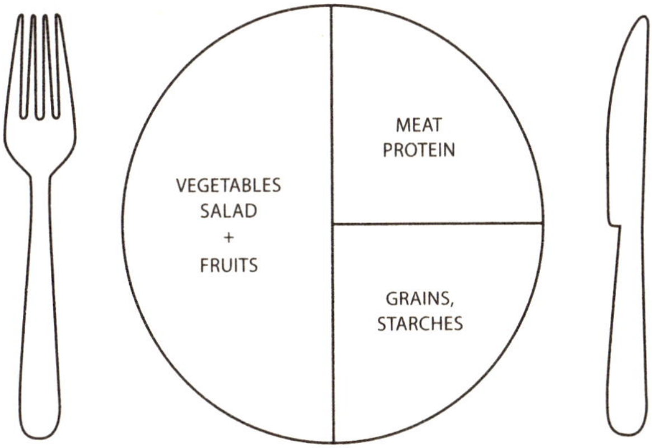

Figure 18: The plate method

Very simply, you take your plate, which may be about 22 centimetres in diameter, and draw an imaginary line down the centre of the plate to divide it into two equal halves. Imagine another line dividing one half into two, as in Figure 18. The plate is now divided into three sections.

Fill the largest portion with non-starchy vegetables such as: salad, spinach, carrots, lettuce, greens, cabbage, green beans, broccoli, cauliflower, tomatoes, onion, cucumber, beets, mushrooms, peppers and root vegetables, like turnips.

In one of the smaller portions put grains and starchy foods. For example:

- wholegrain breads, such as whole wheat or rye
- wholegrain high-fibre cereals, such as bran and grape nuts
- rice, pasta or noodles
- cooked beans and peas, such as pinto beans or black-eyed peas
- potatoes, green peas, corn or sweet potatoes
- low-fat crackers, crisps, pretzels and light popcorn.

A protein, such as those listed below, will occupy the remaining portion on your plate.

- chicken or turkey without the skin
- fish – tuna, salmon, cod, mackerel or sardines
- other seafoods – shrimp, clams, oysters, crab or mussels
- lean cuts of red meat – beef sirloin or pork loin
- tofu, eggs or low-fat cheese.

Add a serving of fruit or a serving of dairy (one cup or 230 millilitres of milk or dairy alternative such as soya or almond milk) or both, to your meal plan.

Generally, only use healthy fats in small amounts. For cooking, use oils. For salads, some healthy additions are nuts, seeds, avocado and vinaigrettes.

Finally, to complete your meal, add a low-calorie drink like water, unsweetened tea or coffee.

Use nature's food bowl

You could say that nature endowed each of us with a food bowl that can be useful in assessing how much food you should have. Basically, cup your hands side-by-side, palms upwards to form a bowl. The total amount of food at any meal should not exceed a slightly heaped natural food bowl. Within that, the protein would be a palmful, while the starches and grains would be equal in size to a fist.

Weight control and Type 2 diabetes

Another of the mainstays of the management of Type 2 diabetes is weight control. Between 80 and 90 per cent of people are overweight when they are first diagnosed with diabetes.

The early death rate of people who are 13.5–18 kilograms overweight is 30 per cent greater than one would expect in a general population of people of normal weight. More alarmingly, there is a 50 per cent increase in early death for men who weigh more than 40 per cent above ideal body weight.

Ideally you should aim for a body mass index (BMI) of between 18.5 and 25. Body mass index is an accepted means of relating weight to height. It is worked out by dividing the weight in kilograms by the square of the height in metres. It is essentially giving an estimation of human body fat, although it does not actually measure fat.

If you need help with weight control then your doctor or practice nurse can advise, or a referral to a dietician can be arranged. Alternatively there are several organisations, like Weight Watchers and Slimming World, which can help in a group situation, wherein you try to lose weight along with other people. The group situation helps many people.

TARGET AND RATE OF WEIGHT LOSS

The target BMI should be 25 or less – the 'healthy' band is 18.5–24.9, and 18.5–22.9 for people of South Asian descent.

For those with a BMI above the healthy range, NICE recommends aiming to achieve weight loss gradually, with a target to reduce weight by five to ten per cent over a period of a year.

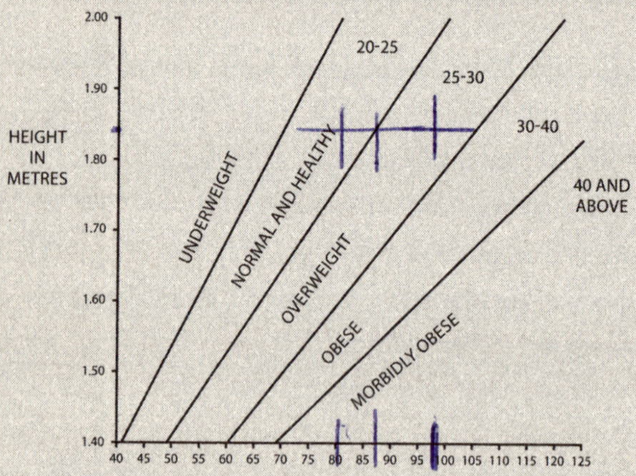

Figure 19: Body mass index for adults

Three keys to weight loss that may surprise you

Recent research suggests that if you want to lose weight there are three key strategies that will increase the chance of success. It seems that if people use these three strategies at once and stick to them, their chance of weight loss increases dramatically. These strategies are simply:

- keep a food journal
- avoid eating out
- do not skip meals.

This research was published in the Journal of the Academy of Nutrition and Dietetics.[21] In this study the researchers investigated a wide range of behaviours and meal patterns in order to find out what worked and what did not. They evaluated changes in body weight of 125 post-menopausal women aged 50–75 years, who were obese, over a study period of one year. The women were divided into a diet only group, a calorie reduction group and a diet plus exercise group. Their average BMI was 31, which categorised them as obese. They all completed questionnaires about what they ate, their meal patterns and food behaviours, such as eating out and keeping food journals and diaries.

After a year the researchers found that all three groups had lost weight, but when they analysed individual behaviours the key strategies seemed to show up quite convincingly. Women who kept a food journal, in which they kept a record of everything they ate every day, lost about 2.7 kilograms more than those who did not. Those who ate regular meals lost on average about 3.6 kilograms more than those who skipped meals. Those who ate out most frequently had the least weight loss. Indeed, even those who ate lunch out once a week lost about 2.2 fewer kilograms than those who never ate out. Fascinatingly, those who used the three key strategies consistently lost the most weight.

These are not, of course, the only things that you should do to lose weight, but they will certainly help the portion control and exercise that you should incorporate into your lifestyle.

TIPS FOR EATING WELL AND STAYING TRIM

1. Eat three regular meals a day and do not skip meals.
2. Eat low-glycaemic, starchy carbohydrates every day – for example: pasta, rice, granary or rye bread, new potatoes, sweet potatoes and porridge.
3. Avoid saturated fats like butter and cheese and use monounsaturated fats like olive oil and rapeseed oil instead.
4. Reduce intake of red meat.
5. Use semi-skimmed or skimmed milk, or non-dairy alternatives like soya, rice or almond milk.
6. Use moist heat to steam, boil and poach as a preferred cooking method.
7. Make sure you have five portions of fruit and vegetables every day and include pulses (lentils, beans and peas).
8. Have three portions of fish, especially oily fish per week – sardines, mackerel, salmon or trout.
9. Reduce salt intake, perhaps using herbs like oregano in place of salt.
10. Restrict sugar and fizzy drinks – look for sugar-free drinks or drink water at meals.
11. Only drink in moderation and have at least two alcohol-free days a week.
12. Use the plate method for portion control.
13. Keep a food diary to monitor what you eat.

Orlistat

If weight loss is a problem then your GP might consider prescribing a drug to help. Orlistat interferes with some of the digestive enzymes that break down fat in the intestines. As a result, about a third of the fat will just pass through you in the bowel motions.

It can produce malodorous motions, loose motions, flatulence and abdominal pains. All of these relate to the undigested fat in the bowel. However, if the fat content of the food is reduced the side effects will settle.

Bariatric surgery

Some people who fall in to the morbid obesity range may be eligible for bariatric surgery if they have:

- found it almost impossible to lose weight on their own.
- not lost weigh despite being prescribed orlistat.
- other medical conditions, like heart disease, that put them at further risk of complications or death.

In the UK, bariatric surgery usually involves gastric banding, although other procedures may be used. None of them are minor operations and the risks have to be measured alongside the benefits.

The Swedish Obesity Study[22] followed up patients who received a variety of operations, including gastric banding. They found that 98 per cent of patients with diabetes had normal blood-glucose levels two years after the operation. However, the long-term results seemed to be best in those patients who had only just developed diabetes. In those who had the condition for several years, although the initial improvement was seen, 70 per cent had reverted to diabetic blood-glucose levels after 15 years.

This should not be viewed negatively, but it emphasises that to maintain a healthy weight you have to adopt good eating habits. Do that and surgery results will be good.

Exercise and Type 2 diabetes

Exercise is one of the mainstays of Type 2 diabetes control. Its benefits are numerous.

- Helps your body use insulin, which controls your blood-sugar
- Burns extra body fat
- Improves blood circulation
- Increases stamina
- Boosts immune system
- Reduces the risk of heart attack
- Reduces the risk of cancers
- Reduces the risk of Alzheimer's disease and other dementias
- Boosts energy and mood
- Strengthens muscles and bones
- Lowers blood pressure
- Cuts LDL (bad) cholesterol
- Raises HDL (good) cholesterol
- Reduces stress.

What sort of exercise

Basically, all exercise is good for you. You do, however, have to check with your GP first to ensure that you are not going to do anything that could prove too much for your heart or which could be problematic if you have high blood pressure. Your GP or diabetic nurse will be able to advise you on suitable exercises.

In the UK, for adults aged 19–64 years, regular exercise is defined by the NHS as completing 150 minutes of moderate-intensity aerobic activity a week. Aerobic activity at moderate intensity basically means exercising at a level that raises your heart rate and makes you perspire. All of the following are suitable exercises.

- Brisk walking
- Light jogging
- Cycling
- Rowing
- Playing doubles tennis or badminton
- Swimming lengths
- Pilates
- Golf.

For older adults over 65 years, who are already fairly fit, they can do the same exercise regime as those in the younger age group. For those less fit, they should discuss with their doctor as to which activities can be safely done according to their level of fitness.

Activities that improve balance and coordination are also worth considering, for example:

- yoga
- t'ai chi
- aquarobics.

NICE also recommend that adults with Type 2 diabetes should undertake muscle strengthening activities for 30–45 minutes, two or three times a week. Your GP can advise you on this.

The NHS has a series of podcasts called the Strength and Flex exercise plan. This is a five-week programme available online and can be downloaded to your computer (see Directory of useful addresses: Get Fit with Stretch and Flex).

Take care if you are on prescribed medication for your Type 2 diabetes. You should take precautions if you take insulin or oral diabetes medication, like sulphonylureas, as exercise may lower your blood-glucose and there is then a risk of hypoglycaemia. This is something to discuss with your GP.

- If your blood-sugar level is less than 5.5 mmol/l (100 mg/dl) prior to exercise, take a carbohydrate snack before beginning the exercise.
- If your blood-sugar level is higher than 5.5 mmol/l (100 mg/dl) before exercise, it may not be necessary to take a carbohydrate snack before a light exercise session, but you may need extra carbohydrates during or following the exercise. Check your blood to see if your blood-sugar dips below 4.0 mmol/l (70 mg/dl) following exercise.
- If you experience hypoglycaemia, check with your doctor. You may need to lower your medication on days you exercise.

- For long duration and high intensity exercise sessions, plan extra carbohydrate snacks during the activity.
- Additional carbohydrates are suggested each 30–60 minutes of exercise. You should consider this if playing football, squash or tennis or going for a long walk or cycle ride.
- Always carry a fast-acting carbohydrate food, such as glucose tablets, when exercising in the event blood-sugar drops too low and hypoglycaemia symptoms develop during exercise.
- You should wear a form of ID, which identifies you as having diabetes, particularly if you are exercising alone so that others may help you appropriately in the event that something unexpected happens.

MEDICALERT ID JEWELLERY

You can obtain discs, bracelets, necklaces and watches, which have the details of your condition and treatment inscribed on them. They help make sure that you receive fast, relevant treatment in an emergency.

Worn on your pulse point, they carry the international medical symbol and are an effective way to communicate vital details to any doctor seeing you in an emergency (see Directory of useful addresses).

Do not forget the non-sport exercises

There are other exercises that may not cause you to break into a sweat, but which are still good for you.

- Housework

- Gardening
- Raking leaves
- Bowling
- Walking and strolling
- Ballroom or other dancing
- Chair aerobics
- Shopping and carrying groceries.

There have been several studies that show the benefits of housework as a form of mild exercise. It can reduce the risk of diabetes and heart disease. Research from Indiana University in the USA shows that adults with high blood pressure may be able to lower their blood pressure with tasks like raking leaves, going for brisk walks and doing housework. Effectively, cumulative activities like these have a profound activity on the circulation.

Stop smoking

NHS Stop Smoking Services offer support that works. You are up to four times more likely to quit smoking successfully if you go to your local NHS Stop Smoking Service and use stop smoking medicines, than if you try to quit using willpower alone.

They can help you with:

- strategies
- chewing gums
- nicotine patches
- drugs – bupropion (Zyban) and varenicline (Champix).

Chapter 9

Drugs for Type 2 diabetes

If diet, weight control and increased activity are not achieving control of the blood-glucose, then medication may be needed. Usually this will be in the form of tablets. It may be that one drug will be needed, but many people need to have a combination of various drugs, also in tablet form. If the combination fails to control blood-glucose then insulin by regular injections or other medication that is also given in injectable form may be needed. I will run through the various drugs that may be used in Type 2 diabetes.

Metformin

This is usually the first drug to be used in Type 2 diabetes. It belongs to the biguanide group of drugs, of which it is the only one used in practice.

It works by:

- stopping the liver from releasing glucose into the bloodstream.
- stimulating the cells of the body to be more sensitive to insulin, that is, it is an insulin sensitiser.

It is a particularly good drug for those who have a weight problem because unlike some of the other drugs, it tends not to encourage further weight gain. In part, this is because it can reduce appetite. Metformin can be prescribed once, twice or three times a day, either with or after a meal. An extended release form, which controls how fast the drug is released, is also available.

Possible side effects include:

- nausea
- vomiting
- diarrhoea
- decreased vitamin B12 absorption.

Metformin can interact with alcohol, so if someone is on this drug they should not drink alcohol.

It should not be used if the person has kidney impairment, since it can cause a dangerous condition called lactic acidosis (see Chapter 7: *The complications of diabetes*).

Sulphonylureas

This is the name of another group of drugs. They work by stimulating the pancreas to secrete insulin from the beta cells of the islets of Langerhans (see the section on insulin and glucagon in Chapter 3: *Metabolism and what goes wrong in diabetes*). They can be taken once or twice a day and they are prescribed if the person cannot take metformin or if weight is not an issue. They do have a tendency to make the person gain weight. They can be used in combination with metformin.

The following are commonly used examples of the sulphonylurea group: glibenclamide, gliclazide, glimepiride, glipizide and gliquidone.

Possible side effects are:

- nausea
- diarrhoea
- weight gain
- hypoglycaemia – low blood-sugar.

DEALING WITH HYPOGLYCAEMIA

- Mild hypoglycaemia can be dealt with by eating or drinking approximately 10–20 grams of sugar (that is, carbohydrates). If you are on a sulphonylurea tablet it is a good idea to carry glucose tablets in case of this.
- Serious hypoglycaemia – when the person becomes drowsy and may lose consciousness – requires urgent medical attention. A GP or paramedic will use an injection of glucagon into the thigh or arm or provide glucose intravenously.

Glitazones

The glitazones, or thiazolidenediones to use their correct name, are a relatively new group of drugs for the treatment of Type 2 diabetes. They work by helping the body to use the insulin that it produces more effectively. Rather like metformin, they sensitise the body to its own insulin. They are used in combination with metformin or the sulphonylureas, or with both. They are not used on their own, but added in when control is being hard to achieve. They can be taken once or twice a day.

Pioglitazone is the drug from this group that is used. Another one called rosiglitazone was withdrawn in 2010 because of an increased risk of heart attack and of heart failure.

Possible side effects of pioglitazone:

- weight gain
- fluid retention
- heart failure in people with co-existing heart disease
- increased risk of bone fractures.

Acarbose

This is an alpha-glucosidase inhibitor, which means that it inhibits a specific enzyme in the small intestine lining. It slows down the rate at which carbohydrates are broken down into glucose. It has to be taken at the start of a meal, since it has to be at the site of its action at the same time as the carbohydrates. It is prescribed infrequently, but is added when control with a combination of drugs is proving difficult.

Possible side effects of acarbose:

- bloating
- diarrhoea
- abdominal pains
- skin rashes.

Incretin therapy

We considered the incretin hormones in Chapter 3 (*Metabolism and what goes wrong in diabetes*). There are two of these hormones:

- glucagon-like peptide 1 (GLP-1)
- glucose-dependent insulinotropic polypeptide (GIP).

They are produced from small glands within the small intestine and their purpose is to:

- stimulate the production of insulin after you eat.
- reduce the production of glucagon by the liver during digestion when it is not needed.
- slow digestion.
- decrease appetite.

These hormones are quickly cleared from the bloodstream by an enzyme called dipeptidyl peptidase (DPP-4).

In people with Type 2 diabetes whose glucose levels are not controlled with the first-line drugs of metformin, sulphonylureas or glitazones, then incretin therapy might help.

There are two approaches:

- inhibit the enzyme that clears these hormones from the body with gliptins, or
- mimic the effect of incretin with drugs called incretin mimetics (GLP-1 agonists).

1. Gliptins – DPP-4 inhibitors

These stop the enzyme DPP-4 from breaking down the incretin, GLP-1. They help to stop the high blood-glucose levels. They are used if a person has not responded to a combination or if he or she cannot use sulphonylureas or glitazones. They can also be used in addition to the other drugs.

The gliptin group includes sitagliptin, vildagliptin and saxagliptin.

They do not cause weight gain, because they reduce appetite and they do not cause hypoglycaemia. They are given orally by mouth.

Possible side effects:

- nausea
- diarrhoea
- abdominal pains
- headache
- nasal congestion
- sore throat
- skin rashes
- pancreatitis (inflammation of the pancreas).

2. Incretin mimetics – GLP-1 agonists

These are drugs that mimic the effect of the incretin hormone GLP-1. They are given by injection to boost insulin production. There are two drugs used in this group: liraglutide, given by injection once a day, and exenatide, which is given by injection twice a day. There is also a form of exenatide that can be given once a week.

These drugs are usually reserved for people who are obese and who have not responded to oral medication. There is some evidence that they help with weight loss. Hypoglycaemia is unlikely with them.

Possible side effects of incretin mimetics:

- nausea
- loss of appetite
- vomiting
- diarrhoea
- headaches
- dizziness
- indigestion
- constipation.

Glinides

These are prandial glucose regulators. This means that they are used to affect blood-glucose levels at meal times. They are taken by mouth, half an hour before meals, three times a day. They are not frequently prescribed as they can cause weight gain and hypoglycaemia.

There are two drugs used: nateglinide and repaglinide.

Gliflozins

These are the sodium-glucose co-transporter-2 (SGLT2) inhibitors. They are a new group of oral medications used for treating Type 2 diabetes. They work by stopping the kidneys from reabsorbing glucose back into the bloodstream. The excess glucose is passed in the urine.

The group includes: dapagliflozin and canagliflozin.

They are suitable for people with Type 2 diabetes who have high blood-glucose levels despite being on drugs like metformin and insulin.

They are not suitable for people with nephropathy, since diminished kidney function will prevent the drug from working.

Possible side effects:

- increased urine output.
- increased tendency to urinary infections and thrush because of the excess glucose in the urine.
- urine testing will not be suitable for managing the condition, since there will always be glucose in the urine.

Insulin therapy

If drug treatment with the oral medications considered above has not worked, then insulin may be needed.

In Type 1 diabetes several types of insulin (long-acting, medium-acting and short-acting) can be used, so the person may need several injections a day.

In Type 2 diabetes if insulin is needed, long-acting insulin is usually given as a single dose at bedtime.

If you are prescribed insulin, then regular blood-glucose monitoring is necessary and your GP will advise about hypoglycaemia and how to recognise and control it and how to adjust the dosage used.

KEY POINTS

SIDE EFFECTS AND DRUG INTERACTIONS

- Always read the leaflet that accompanies any prescription. This will give a full list of cautions and side effects.
- Drug interactions – some of these drugs can interact with alcohol or over-the-counter drugs. Always check with your pharmacist before buying drugs for other conditions like colds or pain relief.

Other drug treatment

This is not treatment of the diabetes, but the treatment of other conditions that may complicate or coexist with the diabetes.

Hypertension

This is commonly present. Drug treatment will be required if there is evidence of end organ damage from hypertension. For example, changes in the retina of the eye or indication of kidney damage.

There are three main groups of drugs used in the treatment of hypertension. These are:

- angiotensin-converting enzyme (ACE inhibitors) or angiotensin receptor blockers (ARBs)
- calcium channel blockers
- diuretics.

About half of people treated with drugs need two or three types of drugs. If a combination of drugs from the above groups of drugs is not tolerated or if they are not controlling the blood pressure, then the following drug groups may be added:

- beta blockers
- alpha blockers.

ACE inhibiters and ARB inhibitors

ACE inhibitors work by dilating the blood vessels to reduce blood pressure and enhance blood flow. ACE inhibitors and ARB inhibitors are important drug groups for people with Type 2 diabetes who have hypertension, especially if they also have nephropathy. They may reduce the risk of further kidney damage.

The most commonly used ACE inhibitors are lisinopril, perindopril, captopril, ramipril and enalapril. Captopril is the oldest and has to be taken twice a day, whereas the others have only to be used once daily.

ACE inhibitors do have some side effects. The most troublesome one is a dry irritant cough. They also cause:

- dizziness
- low blood pressure
- disorder kidney function
- increased risk of ankle swelling.

ARB inhibitors work in a similar way to ACE inhibitors by widening blood vessels and reducing blood pressure. They may be prescribed instead of ACE inhibitors because they do not usually cause a cough.

Commonly used ARBs include candesartan, losartan, telmisartan and valsartan.

They do also have side effects (although not as often a ACE inhibiters) including:

- low blood pressure, which may cause dizziness.
- high levels of potassium in the blood. It is for this reason that your doctor will carry out regular blood tests to monitor the potassium.

Raised lipids

Patients with Type 2 diabetes have an increased risk of heart disease and of having a heart attack, so it is important to have lipid levels done. If these are raised, then statins or other lipid-lowering drugs may be needed.

When blood is taken for lipids, the GP measures three types of fat:

- high-density lipoprotein (HDL)
- low-density lipoprotein (LDL)
- triglycerides.

Statins

Statins can reduce mortality from heart disease by about one third so are invaluable drugs. They are the drugs of first choice in reducing cholesterol levels by up to 40 per cent. They do this by reducing the production of cholesterol in the liver.

The statins, or HMG-CoA reductase inhibitors, have been used for several years to reduce cholesterol levels. They work by inhibiting the enzyme HMG-CoA reductase, which is involved in cholesterol synthesis. The statins work to reduce the level of the enzyme in the liver, which will result in a decrease in the level of cholesterol. They also increase the synthesis of LDL receptors, which helps them to clear low-density lipoproteins from the blood.

Commonly used statins are: atorvastain, fluvastatin, pravatsatin, simvastatin and rosuvastatin.

Possible side effects of statins:

- Some people react to statins and develop muscle cramps and an inflammatory condition of the muscles called a myopathy. At its extreme form it can cause a breakdown in muscle tissue, called rhabdomyolysis.
- Nerve damage is also a rare possibility
- Hair loss
- Nausea
- Abdominal pains
- Pancreatitis
- Altered liver function.

Yet having said that, most people tolerate statins and if one statin produces side effects then another in the group may well be tolerated well.

Fibrates

Fibrates are another type of lipid-lowering drug. They are used for reducing triglyceride levels.

Commonly used fibrates are: bezafibrate, ciprofibrate and fenofibrate.

Both statins and fibrates will be used in combination if there is difficulty in reducing both cholesterol and triglycerides.

Stroke and heart attack prevention with aspirin

The use of aspirin in stroke and heart attack prevention is controversial. At one time, all people with Type 2 diabetes were advised to take aspirin, provided there were no complications. However, the POPADAD trial, the Prevention of Progression of Arterial Disease and Diabetes, did not find any specific evidence that aspirin prevented arterial disease in diabetes.[23]

Having said that, if the person is known to have evidence of hardening of the arteries or is known to be at increased risk of heart attack or stroke, then it is reasonable to take aspirin in a low dose of 75 milligrams daily. That is a quarter of the usual aspirin dose. You should not self-medicate, but only take this after discussion with your GP. Aspirin has lots of potential side effects.

You should *never* take aspirin if you:

- have a history of stomach ulceration.
- have a history of asthma.
- have had a haemorrhagic stroke.
- have any blood disorder or inherited condition, which could predispose you to bleeding.

- have had an allergic reaction to aspirin at any time in your life. There would be the danger of having an anaphylactic reaction, which is a serious, potentially life-threatening allergic reaction characterised by low blood pressure, shock and difficulty breathing. It is a medical emergency.
- are under 16 years of age.
- are on drugs like anticoagulants, or other drugs that could interact with aspirin to increase the risk of a bleed.

Diabetic kidney disease

As mentioned above, an angiotensin-converting enzyme (ACE) inhibitor, such as enalapril, lisinopril or ramipril, should be prescribed if there are early signs of diabetic kidney disease. This is shown to reduce the risk of further damage.

Chapter 10

Using the Life Cycle with Type 2 diabetes

'Do not dwell in the past, do not dream of the future, concentrate the mind on the present moment.' Buddha

In my own practice I use a model that I call the Life Cycle to help patients to examine their life in order to devise strategies that they can use for self-help. I do not pretend that this is any kind of rocket science. It is simply a model that many people find useful in gaining a bit of focus.

The Life Cycle

This term 'life cycle' may take you back to your days of studying biology when you looked at the different life cycles of insects, fish, frogs and other creatures on the evolutionary ladder. I am not, however, using the term here in the same sense. I am using it as a model for a person's life. This has nothing to do with his or her development with age, but is to do with the different levels or spheres that make up one's life at any point in time. You will see that there is a cycle involved, certainly in the manner in which a condition – virtually any chronic medical condition, whether that is a physical one or a psychological one like depression – can affect them.

Yet to use the biology analogy a little longer, you will learn a certain amount about fish by dissecting them to look at their internal organs, but you will not know how they move and feed without studying them in water, and you will not learn about their behaviour with other fish and predators unless you observe them in a realistic environment. Even then you will not get to know about them fully unless you just become a total observer of them.

So it is in medicine. In order to help someone you need to know as much as possible about his or her condition, symptoms and the things that make symptoms better or worse. And ideally you want to know about his or her habits, diet, desires, fears, relationships and so on. That might seem like a tall order, but if you can build up such a picture of the patient, then you can see how a condition is truly affecting him or her throughout all levels of his or her life.

This is what you need to do in order to help yourself manage a condition in the most effective way that you can. This model enables the individual to build a picture of his or her life and the way the different spheres of that life interact in a cyclical manner.

There are five levels or spheres of life that we need to consider.

1. Body – what are the physical symptoms? Is there pain, stiffness or tiredness, for example?

2. Emotions – how you feel? Are you anxious, sad, depressed, angry or jealous of others?

3. Mind – what type of thoughts do you have? Are they pessimistic thoughts, negative thoughts, self-defeating thoughts, happy thoughts or optimistic thoughts?
4. Behaviour – how does the condition or symptom make you behave? For example, are you isolating yourself by avoiding things or people or developing habits like smoking, drinking or becoming inactive?
5. Lifestyle – how does the condition or symptom affect your ability to do things and your relationships? How do events in your life impact on you?

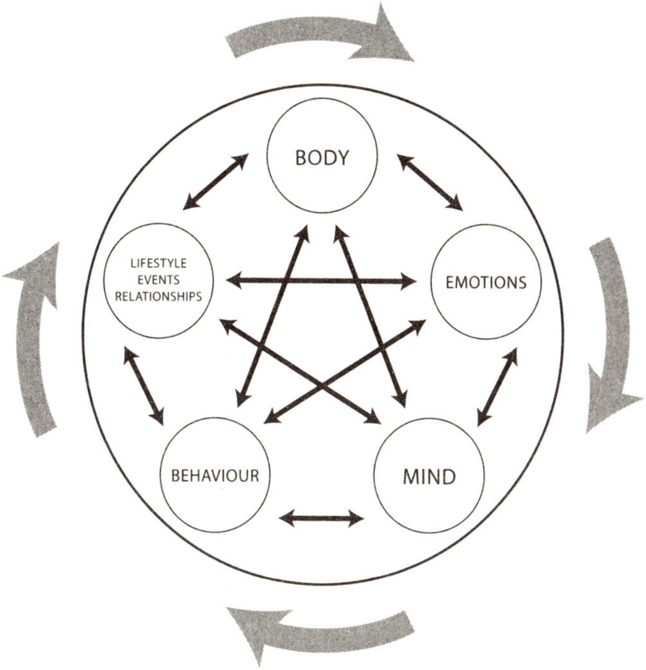

Figure 20: The Life Cycle

Now take a look at Figure 20. You will see the five spheres starting with the 'Body' sphere at the top. If you follow the direction of the large arrows you will see that it follows the order above – body, emotions, mind, behaviour and lifestyle. Note that the outer circle that encloses the whole structure. This represents the individual's whole self, his or her life. In other words, the five spheres all make up part of the individual's experience of life.

The five double-headed arrows sitting just inside the circle represent the general progression, the Life Cycle, because the order represents the way that a physical condition will tend to impact on a person. That is, a physical condition and physical symptoms make the individual aware that something is wrong in the body. This can induce an emotional response, which could be anxiety, anger, resentment or fear. The emotions felt alter the way that you think and the type of thoughts that you have. This may make you take a particular action or to behave in a way: reach for a drink, order a beef burger, take a tablet or avoid a situation. Your actions or behaviours may affect your lifestyle, stopping you from doing things that may affect relationships and work. And all of that can set the cycle off again.

The six double-headed arrows in the centre of the circle show that every sphere impacts on every single other one. A pain, for example, impacts on all spheres of your life. On the other hand, the inner arrows give you the opportunity to use any of the other spheres to modify or deal better with a problem.

The same thing goes if your starting point is not a physical symptom, but the way that you feel. Anxiety, for example, can be looked at in exactly the same way. It is felt in the emotional sphere. It makes you think in a particular way, which makes you tend to act in a particular way and it will impact on your lifestyle. You may or may not feel physical symptoms. Looking at the inner arrows you have lots of potential ways that by improving one sphere you can affect your anxiety. It may not give a magical result, but if you can break the chain, use alternative pathways, you can devise strategies that will help you to cope.

In the case of low spirits or mild depression, if you realise that you do not have to keep repeating the same cycle which basically locks you into feeling down, then you start to reduce the feeling of hopelessness that tends to go hand in hand with depression. Once you start to break the cycle and prove that you are not helpless and that the situation is not hopeless your spirits may rise.

It is not a case of feeling low and telling yourself to 'pull your socks up' as that very rarely works; instead it is a means of getting your mind to work for you by getting in to a different pattern of thinking.

Develop positive thinking

If you are of a pessimistic nature then you are more likely to become depressed, feel anxious, experience more pain and even have a higher risk of conditions like heart disease and cerebrovascular disease. You are also more likely to pick up colds and other respiratory infections.

It is thought that this is in part due to a psycho-neuro-immunological (PNI) mechanism. This refers to the growing realisation that the mind (psyche), the nervous system (neuro) and the immune system are all interconnected. Thus stress can affect the nervous system and thence the immune system. A lot of stress can throw a strain on the whole system, so that the immune system works below par and one can pick up an infection.

We all operate these PNI mechanisms to varying degrees and you can have positive PNI mechanisms and negative ones. A positive one is seen in people who are able to delay an illness, but who may then go down with something on the first day of their holiday. A negative one is seen when some stress is immediately followed by an illness. This can take one out of the work environment. Pessimists are more likely to operate the negative PNI mechanisms and optimists the positive ones.

The essence of all this is that we have a choice as to how we view things. One must work against a tendency to be pessimistic and to try to become an optimist. To begin with, you have to consider self-talk. This is the name that is given to the endless stream of thoughts that run through our head every day. Pessimists, who may be more prone to anxiety and depression, tend to have a lot of negative automatic thought. Let me give you four examples of such negative thought.

- Filtering – is where the individual filters out all the positives and sees only the negative. For example, despite a good day at work, he or she focuses on the single error.
- Personalisation – whenever something goes wrong he or she automatically assumes it is his or her fault.
- Catastrophising – the individual extrapolates all situations to the worst scenario, usually finding a reason for not doing something to prevent a supposed humiliation risk.
- Polarisation – the person sees everything as two poles, good or bad, black or white, with nothing between.

To think positively, you have to monitor your self-talk and try to alter the negativity. Instead of thinking 'I can't do it because I have never done it before,' try thinking, 'It's an opportunity to learn.' Or instead of 'There is no way this will work for me,' try 'Let me attempt to make this work.'

This is all very relevant to the Life Cycle, because if you allow yourself to become pessimistic then you will get into a particular mindset. You will affect your emotions and tend to get anxious and depressed. This in turn will make you tend to adopt particular behaviour patterns.

Returning to the example of pain. If you anticipate that you are going to have a pain, you may end up taking more painkillers, and you may end up taking them when you do not actually need them. An optimist, on the other hand, may feel that the pain will go away if he or she does something else. That is, adopt another behaviour pattern that will distract from the pain, which as we have seen can make matters easier.

Logotherapy

Let me tell you about this quite remarkable therapy, which was developed by a remarkable man. I first came across it when I was working in psychiatry at the start of my medical career.

Viktor Frankl was the founder of a system of psychiatry known as Logotherapy. This is sometimes referred to as the 'Third Viennese School of Psychiatry'. Sigmund Freud's psychoanalysis is accepted as being the first, and Alfred Adler's Individual Psychology was the second. Frankl had developed his theories during stays in three concentration camps, including the dreaded Auschwitz.

In establishing his philosophy of Logotherapy, Frankl established three basic beliefs. Firstly, that life has meaning under all circumstances, even the most miserable ones. Secondly, that our main motivation is our will to find meaning in life. Thirdly, that we have freedom to find meaning in what we do and what we experience.

One of Frankl's key concepts was that of anticipatory anxiety. This is actually more than simply the fear that one has before an event. It is the anxiety about something happening, which actually is more likely to make it happen. For example, for someone with insomnia, the worry that he or she won't sleep is often so great that he or she probably will not sleep.

The aim of Logotherapy is to change the attitude towards how one feels about life and to remove that important anticipatory fear. In Logotherapy a technique of paradoxical intention is used instead.

Taking the example of insomnia. People troubled with it usually go to bed and try too hard to sleep, the result being that they cannot sleep. With paradoxical intention you try to do the exact opposite. That is, you go to bed and you try 'not to sleep'. You may be amazed at how hard it then is to stay awake.

Another example is during a hiccup attack. Instead of trying to stop them, try to make yourself hiccup. Offer yourself ten pounds to hiccup again. This paradoxical intention method usually makes them just stop.

Let us look at some situations that are very common in Type 2 diabetes.

Despondency and negative emotions in Type 2 diabetes

These can occur very often and may be triggered by a definite event, such as a consultation with the GP or diabetic nurse, or the blood-glucose measurements may seem to have gone out of control.

This may lower the mood and make the person feel despondent about the condition, about the management of the diabetes and induce anxiety about the future.

The thoughts that the person may have could be like these:

- Why has this happened to me (the diabetes)?
- What have I done to deserve this?
- Controlling this is too difficult!
- Whatever I do will not help!
- I have this chronic disease for the rest of my life!
- Oh, what's the use!

The emotions could be:

- anger at the condition.
- resentment that other members of the family do not have to control their diets.
- guilt that others will not think you are doing your best.
- despondency.
- irritability towards everyone.
- frustration that the condition or symptom is not settling.

The behaviour could be:

- giving up on the diet.
- denying that there is a problem.
- being contrary and doing the opposite of what you know is best, perhaps bingeing.

- avoiding exercise.
- avoiding weighing yourself.
- avoiding doing blood-glucose measurements.
- only looking after yourself in a half-hearted manner.

The lifestyle effects could be:

- the adoption of habits that could affect your condition.
- relationship issues can result because of increased irritability, anger, depression or frustration.

It may be helpful to sketch out your Life Cycle diagram on a piece of paper, jotting down the thoughts, emotions, actions and lifestyle entries. Also note any physical symptoms or otherwise. Look at the arrows on Figure 20 and give some thought to ways that the different spheres interact. The aim is then to think about how modifying one can modify the other and impact on how you feel and how you think. For example:

Mind
Go to the thoughts sphere and challenge the thoughts.

- Controlling it is not too difficult. Hundreds of thousands of people control their diabetes.
- Whatever I do will have an effect!
- I just have to infuse positive thinking into the equation.

Behaviour

You can certainly change the behaviour.

- I am not giving up on the diet.
- I am not an ostrich; I will not stick my head in the sand.
- I am going to exercise and I am going to see the benefit.

Lifestyle

Lifestyle effects can be modified.

- Being irritable is rude and hurtful to those I love; I will not be rude.
- I am going to show the family that I can brighten everyone's life.

You see, you can develop strategies to help. By visualising them and drawing the Life Cycle you can see the map of your life and you can see different ways to modify the journey to wellness.

Chronic pain

We saw in Chapter 7 (*The complications of diabetes*) that neuropathy or nerve damage can lead to chronic pain or to chronic paraesthesia (pins and needles). One of the problems in this sort of situation is that pain or pins and needles that persist with little respite (which we call chronic pain as opposed to acute pain that is limited and will eventually end) is that it is relayed to the brain in a different manner from short-lived pain.

This has been demonstrated by recent research from the Northwestern University's Feinberg School of Medicine in Chicago. Using functional Magnetic Resonance Imaging (fMRI) scans of people with pain problems the researchers were actually able to demonstrate that acute and chronic pain light up different parts of the brain.

In acute pain, such as occurs with a burned finger or an acute muscle strain, there is intense activity within the thalamus in the midbrain. By contrast, chronic pain lights up the prefrontal cortex at the front of the brain and the limbic system. The prefrontal cortex is involved in higher thought processing, and the limbic system is part of the brain that seems to be involved in emotions.

They also found that the longer a person has been experiencing chronic pain the more activity occurs in the prefrontal cortex. This rather implies that the brain then holds a memory of the pain that can keep being replayed. It also implies that the emotional aspect of the pain will tend to be replayed.

The significance of this is that drugs are not necessarily going to solve the problem of a chronic painful condition. They may suppress parts of the perception of the pain, yet they will do nothing for that part which is laid down as a memory trace, or which has an emotional memory. This very much fits in with the experience of people who have developed a chronic pain problem.

The human pain matrix

This is the current concept of pain perception. It is thought that there is a matrix, or a whole network of ways that nerve impulses can be passed up to the brain, which perceives the pain. This matrix seems to have two main components in the brain, which operate in parallel with each other.

1. The lateral pain system seems to be responsible for processing the physical sensations, such as intensity of pain and its localization. It has much to do with acute pain such as the pain you feel when part of the body is traumatised.

2. The medial pain system processes the emotional side of pain. It passes its information up medially. And it does it through the limbic system. The information is then passed up to the prefrontal cortex.

The Life Cycle and chronic pain

As we have just seen, chronic pain will probably have an emotional content, and as a result of the emotional memory being triggered it may well be associated with a particular chain of thoughts that come to mind. Thus, the pain triggers the emotion of anxiety – 'Oh dear, here is that awful pain again. The only thing to do is to take a painkiller.'

In other words, a negative emotion and a negative thought and the resultant behaviour is triggered. This is not to say that the action of taking a painkiller is a negative behaviour. It may be the right thing to do, but it is not always the right thing to do.

If instead of allowing the negative emotion and the negative thought to come to the fore, if the individual can think a positive thought, such as 'the pain will go away soon,' at the same time reflecting on a happy image or event and doing something totally different, like pruning the roses, starting a crossword or making a cup of tea, then the action of taking a painkiller may not be needed or acted upon.

Success begets success and if this distraction works once it will work again, and this method can be used to focus on the whole situation or upon any symptom or behaviour that you would like to modify.

Try using the imagination as a painkiller

Some years ago I attended a very interesting photographic exhibition at St Thomas' Hospital in London. The theme was chronic pain. I thought it was an extremely clever idea because it introduced an artistic perspective to the enigma of pain.

The photographs in the exhibition were portrayals of people's perceptions of their pain. One photograph showed a concrete straitjacket that the artist had made to illustrate one person's experience and perception of their pain. To that person pain was a solid thing, a constricting and isolating thing, and it weighed him or her down, just as concrete would.

Other images showed red-hot wires glowing in the dark, animal scratches on stone and gloves full of crawling ants. You can imagine the quality of the pain those people were experiencing. It is really interesting, because no two people experience the same pain. It has a unique feel and, if you think about the concept of the pain matrix, there is a unique blend of emotions associated with it.

The imagery that one can use to describe a pain therefore gives you a means of using your imagination as a painkiller. When you have a pain try to imagine what your pain looks like in a symbolic manner. Try to get your own picture of it rather than thinking of how severe it is.

If you can do that then you can modify the image and by doing that you can reduce the actual level of pain. For example, if you have a pain in your back that feels like a tight band or a taut rope, then close your eyes and visualise that rope with a great big tight knot in it. Focus hard and mentally try to loosen the knot.

You may feel the pain as though it is burning like a smouldering rope. Hold that picture in your mind, and imagine the pain getting less intense as the rope is soaked in water, until the burning is totally extinguished.

Peripheral neuropathy may produce a glove and stocking distribution of numbness, pain or pins and needles. Using your imagination, envisage that you actually are wearing gloves or stockings that are under your control. You can make the gloves or stockings heat up, cool down, become less sensitive or whatever helps lessen the pain.

Use your imagination to remedy whatever picture your mind conjures. A cold pain like an icicle could be warmed and melted by imagining it being gently heated. A boring corkscrew-like pain could be gently unwound from a cork.

So try it the next time you have pain. Sit or lie down somewhere you will not be disturbed and make yourself as comfortable as possible. Let your mind throw up images that seem appropriate, and when you have the image that corresponds best with the pain, use your mind to reverse the effect. As you do this, tell yourself that you are reducing the pain, lessening the discomfort until it goes.

Your imagination is very powerful. It can make you feel emotional, so it makes perfect logic to get it to work for you. You can affect the medial pain system that controls the emotional component of pain. You can use it as a painkiller. Try doing this for 20 minutes every day for a week.

Sexual problems

As mentioned in Chapter 7 (*The complications of diabetes*), many people experience loss of libido. This can occur as a result of psychological factors or physical ones, such as increased tendency to thrush, physical discomfort due to lack of lubrication, altered sensation or a hormonal imbalance taking away the desire. If there is a problem, then see your GP to exclude a physical cause or to see if there is any treatment that will improve matters.

Yet, using the Life Cycle method you may be able to help matters alone or with your partner.

Lack of libido can result in a range of emotions:

- guilt
- irritability
- frustration
- low mood
- anxiety.

These can lead to various behaviours:

- avoidance of sex
- irritability, as an unconscious mechanism to fend off your partner
- overindulgence in alcohol
- overindulgence in food
- smoking
- taking recreational drugs
- gambling.

In other words, people can use other unconscious psychological mechanisms to compensate for their lack of libido. In turn, this can have an effect on lifestyle, since it can affect the relationship with one's partner.

You can again sketch out the Life Cycle and be honest and jot down what occurs to you for each of the spheres. Then you can challenge the beliefs that you have developed around the thoughts, the emotions and the actions. By concentrating on the inner arrows and the different spheres you can find ways of breaking the cycle.

In general, mutual discussion between partners can remove anxiety. Both partners may have interpreted the lack of libido in different ways that may both affect the relationship. For example, one partner may feel that the loss of libido lessens him or her as a person, while the other partner may feel that his or her partner's lack of libido means that he or she no longer finds him or her attractive.

Lack of orgasm, which can be caused by neuropathy, altered hormones or increased anxiety, can also be an issue for some people. It may be that anticipatory anxiety just becomes so great that the whole thought of sex becomes terrifying and the person avoids it at all costs.

Discuss with your partner about whether achieving an orgasm is actually all that important. The process of lovemaking is about mutually pleasuring each other in a loving way. Being patient and being gentle and caring, enjoying caressing and foreplay rather than actual sexual penetration may make the whole act more mutually satisfying.

Erectile dysfunction can result in the same range of emotions as diminished libido. In addition, there is often also considerable anticipatory anxiety.

What usually happens is that after experiencing difficulty achieving an erection on a few occasions the man gets performance anxiety, which itself makes it difficult to achieve an erection. Good counselling will often help, together with a frank discussion between the person with diabetes and their sexual partner.

It may help to know that sexual penetration only needs a 60 per cent erection. Instead of just avoiding sex, talk about it and perhaps agree to put a ban on sexual penetration for a period of time, say a month.

Instead of worrying about whether an erection strong enough for penetration will be achieved, simply indulging in foreplay and possibly oral sex may convince the person that the problem can be overcome. It is important, however, to maintain the ban even if a full erection is achieved, until the length of the ban has run its course. This builds confidence because it totally removes the anticipatory anxiety – the performance anxiety – and allows normal function to take place.

This is a good example of a Logotherapy technique. The simple fact is that if you remove the reason for the anticipatory anxiety by paradoxical intention (see page 207) the anxiety disappears. By not having to perform, the natural erection may well reappear.

Another thing that may help is to consider reading erotica. This is something that affects the behaviour sphere. It is readily available in e-book form from Internet book suppliers and is inexpensive. It is easy to find tasteful erotica, it is totally discreet (since it is viewed with an e-book reader, such as Kindle) and there is no reason whatever to feel guilty. Although you may never have thought of reading such literature, you may find that it does increase your libido and helps you to solve the problem.

It is not all doom and gloom

Receiving the diagnosis that you have Type 2 diabetes is not a reason to become depressed. It is a serious condition, yet it is one that is eminently manageable and when well managed is compatible with a normal life. True, you will probably have to make several changes to your lifestyle, but they are all changes that will result in better health than you were experiencing at the time of diagnosis.

If you are a woman wanting to have a family, your fertility will not be reduced. Your pregnancy should be no more hazardous than your non-diabetic friends and, with good care your baby will be healthy and well.

It is a matter of gaining focus and incorporating good changes into your life. That way you will reduce your risk of the complications that can occur in diabetes. You can and will live well with your Type 2 diabetes.

Glossary

advanced glycation end products, AGEs – these are substances formed in the body when proteins or fats combine with sugars through the process of glycation.

afferent – a blood vessel supplying an organ or tissue.

agonist – a drug given to enhance an effect or to stimulate.

aqueous humour – clear fluid inside the eye, in front of the lens.

arteriosclerosis – hardening of the arteries caused by accumulation of atheroma (same as atherosclerosis).

artery – blood vessel that carries oxygenated blood away from the heart, taking it to specific organs.

aspirin – the common name for acetylsalicylic acid, an anti-platelet agent that thins the blood and may be given to prevent a stroke.

atheroma – fatty changes in a blood vessel.

atherosclerosis – hardening of the arteries caused by accumulation of atheroma.

body mass index, BMI – an accepted means of relating weight to height. It is worked out by dividing the weight in kilograms by the square of the height in metres.

Bowman's capsule – a microscopic structure surrounding the glomerulus in the nephron.

Bruns-Garland's syndrome - another name for proximal motor neuropathy.

Charcot foot – total alteration of the shape of the foot as a result of neuropathy and joint collapse.

cholesterol – a blood lipid or fat. There are two main types LDL cholesterol and HDL cholesterol.

creatinine – a breakdown product of muscle that is excreted in the urine.

efferent – an artery leaving an organ or tissue.

functional Magnetic Resonance Imaging, fMRI – type of MRI scan used on the brain to show brain function during a task.

gastroparesis – damage to the vagus nerve, which supplies the stomach and intestines, may result in impairment of the stomach's ability to empty .

glomerular filtration rate, eGFR – a blood test that assesses how much blood is filtered and cleared of waste products per minute.

glomerulus – a network of blood vessels that forms part of the nephron.

glucagon – a hormone that opposes the action of insulin.

glycation – a process that occurs in the body in which proteins or fats combine with sugars, to produce advanced glycation end products, AGEs.

glycogenesis – the building of glycogen from glucose.

glycolysis – the breaking down of glycogen.

glyconeogenesis – the generation of glucose from non-carbohydrate substances, such as pyruvate, lactate, glycerol and amino acids.

glycosuria – the passage of glucose in the urine.

halitosis – bad breath.

HbA1c – effectively a measure of the blood-glucose levels over the previous two to three months.

Humulin – a medicine used in the treatment of diabetes as a substitute for the body's own insulin.

hyperglycaemia – high blood glucose.

hyperphagia – increased hunger. See also polyphagia.

hypoglycaemia – low blood-glucose.

incretins – hormones produced in the small intestine, needed for the control of blood-glucose at and shortly after meals.

inhibitor – a drug given to reduce a function or to prevent an enzyme from working.

insulin – hormone produced by the pancreas, involved in the control of blood-glucose.

islets of Langerhans – small areas found in the pancreas that produce insulin, glucagon and somastatin, three hormones that regulate the blood-glucose level in the body.

ketoacidosis – a state in which the blood-glucose rises very high and the blood becomes acidic and accumulates ketones.

Krebs cycle – the main energy-producing reaction in the cells.

Kussmaul breathing – deep breathing, or air hunger, in the state of ketoacidosis.

lipogenesis – the building of triglyceride fats from fatty acids.

lipolysis – breaking down fats into fatty acids.

lumen – the space inside a blood vessel through which blood flows.

macroalbuminuria – presence of large amounts of albumin in the urine in diabetic nephropathy and chronic kidney disease.

Magnetic Resonance Imaging (MRI) – a type of scan used in medicine. See also functional Magnetic Resonance Imaging.

meninges – the membranes that cover the brain.

meta-analysis – a statistical technique for combining and analysing the findings of independent trials.

metformin – the most commonly used glucose-lowering drug in Type 2 diabetes.

microalbuminuria – the presence of microscopic amounts of albumin. This is a first sign of early kidney disease.

microhaematuria – the presence of microscopic amounts of blood in the urine, which will not be apparent to the naked eye.

mononeuopathy – a neuropathy affecting a single nerve.

mononeuritis multiplex – neuropathy affecting more than one nerve.

nephron – the microscopic filtering unit of the kidney.

nephropathy – kidney damage.

neuropathy – damage or disease affecting nerves.

NICE – National Institute for Health and Clinical Excellence.

onychomycosis – fungal infection of the nail.

paraesthesia – pins and needles.

polydipsia – increased thirst.

polyphagia – increased appetite.

polyuria – increased frequency of urination.

prandial – relating to meals.

pre-diabetes – a condition when the blood-glucose level is higher than normal, but not high enough to be diagnosed as diabetes. It is a state that increases the risk of diabetes.

prevalence – the number of people with a specific condition at a specified time divided by the total number of people in the population.

proteolysis – breaking down proteins into amino acids.

pyorrhea – pus produced in gum disease.

retina – the light-sensitive 'seeing' membrane at the back of the eyes.

retinal detachment – condition in which the retina peels away from the back of the eyes.

retinopathy – damage to the retina.

septicaemia – a dangerous infection in the blood.

somastatin – a hormone produce by the islets of Langerhans in the pancreas, which inhibits the secretion of the other pancreatic hormones (insulin and glucagon).

statins – a group of drugs used to reduce lipids in the blood.

tubule – part of the nephron, the filtering units of the kidney.

vitrectomy – operation to remove and replace the vitreous humour of the eye.

vitreous humour – jelly-like fluid behind the lenses of the eyes.

WHO – World Health Organization.

References

1 Valdez R. Detecting undiagnosed Type 2 diabetes: family history as a risk factor and screening tool. Journal of Diabetes Science and Technology; (2009) 3: 4, 722-726.

2 UK Prospective Diabetes Study group (1994). UK Prospective Diabetes Study XII. Differences between Asian, Afro Caribbean and White Caucasian Type 2 diabetic patients at diagnosis of diabetes. Diabetic Medicine; 11: 670–167.

3 Danaei G, Finucane MM, Lu Y, Singh GM, Cowan MJ, Paciorek CJ et al. National, regional, and global trends in fasting plasma glucose and diabetes prevalence since 1980: systematic analysis of health examination surveys and epidemiological studies with 370 country-years and 2.7 million participants. Lancet, 2011, 378(9785):31–40.

4 Mathers CD, Loncar D. Projections of global mortality and burden of disease from 2002 to 2030. PLoS Med, 2006, 3(11):e442.

5 2011 Census: Population Estimates for the United Kingdom". Office for National Statistics. 27 March 2011.

6 Singh R, Barden A, Mori T, Beilin L. Advanced glycation end-products: a review, Diabetologia 2001, Volume 44, pp 129–46.

7 Mainous AG, Tanner RJ, Baker R, Zayas CE, Harle CA. Prevalence of pre-diabetes in England from 2003 to 2011: population-based, cross-sectional study BMJ Open 2014;4:e005002. doi:10.1136/bmjopen-2014-005002.

8 Huang Y, Cai X, Qiu M, Chen P, Tang H, Hu Y, Huang Y. Pre-diabetes and the risk of cancer: a meta-analysis. Diabetologia, September 2014 DOI: 10.1007/s00125-014-3361-2.

9 Ashwell M, Gunn P, Gibson N. Waist-to-height ratio is a better screening tool than waist circumference and BMI for adult cardiometabolic risk factors: a systematic review and meta-analysis. Obesity review, 2012, 275–86.

10 McKeown NM, Meigs JB, Liu S, Saltzman E, Wilson PW, Jacques PF. Carbohydrate nutrition, insulin resistance, and the prevalence of the metabolic syndrome in the Framingham Offspring Cohort. Diabetes Care. 2004; 27:538–46.

11 Krishnan S, Rosenberg L, Singer M, et al. Glycemic index, glycemic load, and cereal fiber intake and risk of type 2 diabetes in US black women. Arch Intern Med. 2007; 167:2304–9.

12 Bhupathiraju SN, Pan A, Manson JE, et al. Changes in coffee intake and subsequent risk of type 2 diabetes: three large cohorts of US men and women. Diabetologia. 2014;57:1346–54.

...sociation of glycaemia with macrovascular and microvascular ...ications of Type 2 diabetes: prospective observational study. ...Medical Journal 2000; 321: 405–12.

14 Yudkin JS, Richter B, Gale EA. Intensified glucose lowering in type 2 diabetes: time for a reappraisal. Diabetologia 2010;53:2079–85.

15 Nielsen SF, Nordestgaard B G. Statin use before diabetes diagnosis and risk of microvascular disease: a nationwide nested matched study. Lancet, Volume 2, No. 11, p894–900, 2014.

16 Nielsen SF, Nordestgaard B G. Statin use before diabetes diagnosis and risk of microvascular disease: a nationwide nested matched study. Lancet, Volume 2, No. 11, p894–900, 2014.

17 Dorey G, Speakman MJ, Feneley RCL, Swinkels A. Dunn CDR. Pelvic floor exercises for erectile dysfunction. BJU 2005 Vol 96, pp 595–7.

18 Salas-Salvado J, Bullo M, Babio N, et al. Reduction in the incidence of type 2 diabetes with the Mediterranean diet: results of the PREDIMED-Reus nutrition intervention randomized trial. Diabetes Care. 2011; 34: 14–9.

19 O'Connor LM, Lentjes MAH, Luben RN, Khaw KT, Wareham NJ, Forouhi NG. Dietary dairy product intake and incident type 2 diabetes: a prospective study using dietary data from a 7-day food diary. Diabetologia, 2014; DOI: 10.1007/s00125-014-3176-1.

20 Chen M, Sun Q, Giovannucci E, Mozaffarian D, Manson J.E, Wille WC, Hu FB. Dairy consumption and risk of type 2 diabetes: 3 coh of US adults and an updated meta-analysis. BCM Medicine 12:215.

21 McTiernan A, et al. Self-monitoring and Eating-related Behaviors are Associated with 12-month Weight Loss Among Postmenopausal Overweight-to-obese Women in a Dietary Weight Loss Intervention. Journal of the Academy of Nutrition and Dietetics, 2012.

22 Sjöström L, et al. Effects of bariatric surgery on mortality in Swedish obese subjects. N Engl J Med. 2007 Aug 23;357(8):741-52.

23 Belch J, MacCuish A, Campbell I, et al. The prevention and progression of arterial disease and diabetes (POPADAD) trial: factorial randomised placebo controlled trial of aspirin and antioxidants in patients with diabetes and asymptomatic peripheral arterial disease. BMJ 2008; 337:a1840.